# HOW TO KEEP YOUR
# FEET & LEGS
# HEALTHY
## FOR A LIFETIME

For active parents —

Love,

Noni

October, 1990

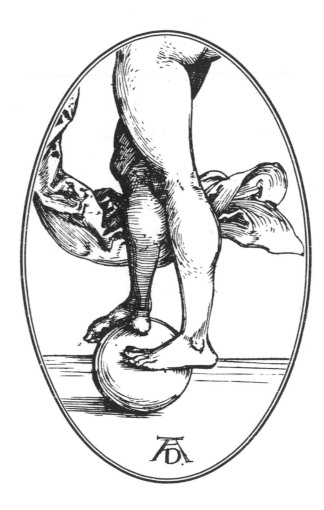

# HOW TO KEEP YOUR
# FEET & LEGS
# HEALTHY
## FOR A LIFETIME

THE ONLY COMPLETE GUIDE
TO FOOT AND LEG CARE
WITH SPECIAL SECTIONS FOR
WALKERS, JOGGERS AND RUNNERS

## BY GARY NULL

### WITH DR. HOWARD ROBINS

FOUR WALLS EIGHT WINDOWS
NEW YORK

Library of Congress Cataloging-in-Publication Data

Null, Gary, 1945–
    How to keep your feet and legs healthy for a lifetime :
the only complete guide to foot and leg care, with sections
for walkers, joggers, and runners / Gary Null, with
Howard Robins. — 1st ed.
      p.  cm.
    ISBN 0-941423-36-0 : $12.95
    1. Foot—Care and hygiene.  2. Leg—Care and
    hygiene.  I. Robins, Howard, 1947-  .  II. Title.
    RD563.N85   1990
    612'.98—dc20                         89-71438
                                                         CIP

Four Walls Eight Windows
P.O. Box 548
Village Station
New York, N.Y. 10014

Printed in the U.S.A.

Cover design by Marty Moskof.

Special thanks to Miranda Ottewell, whose assiduous copyediting made this book possible, and to Naomi Rosenblatt, whose inspired search for illustrative matter brought to these pages images of some of art history's most sublimely beautiful feet.

With special thanks to Gary Null for his encouragement and help, and Trisha Carendi for her help, this book is dedicated to my son Richard, my daughter Jessica and to all the sore feet of the world.

Howard F. Robins, D.P.M.
May, 1990

# CONTENTS

The Benefits of a Walking Program, 99.
Special Advice for Heart Patients, 100.
Other Special Situations, 101.

## 7 FOOTWEAR 103

BUYING A SHOE, 105.  Fit, 105.
Materials and Construction, 107.  Style, 108.
SHOES FOR WORK, 111.
SHOES FOR SPORTS, 112.  Running, Jogging,
and Walking, 113.  Racquet Sports, 119.
Basketball, 120.  Baseball, 120.  Boating, 120.
Roller Skating, 121.  Cycling, 122.  Golf, 122.
Weight Lifting, 123.  Wrestling and Boxing, 123.
Fencing, 124.  SOCKS FOR SPORTS, 124.
ORTHOTIC DEVICES, 126.
Orthotic Devices for Children, 130.

## 8 MASSAGE 133

BENEFITS OF MASSAGE, 136.
THE TEN-MINUTE MORNING MASSAGE, 137.
IN-DEPTH FOOT AND LEG MASSAGE, 139.

APPENDIX A: AN ANATOMICAL FRAMEWORK 143

APPENDIX B:
HERBAL SOLUTION AND SALVE RECIPES 151

APPENDIX C:
SUPPLIERS OF FOOTWEAR PRODUCTS 155

GLOSSARY 159

# ILLUSTRATIONS

# ANATOMICAL DRAWINGS

For the want of a nail, the shoe was lost.
For the want of a shoe, the horse was lost.
For the want of a rider, the battle was lost.
For the want of a battle, the kingdom was lost—
and all for the want of a horseshoe nail!

—Benjamin Franklin *Poor Richard's Almanac*

# HOW TO KEEP YOUR
# FEET & LEGS
# HEALTHY
## FOR A LIFETIME

# INTRODUCTION

A CONSUMER REVOLUTION is transforming health care today. Millions of people are no longer satisfied to be passive consumers of medical services: they don't trust the medical profession to always know what's best for them. They want to understand their bodies so that they can take responsibility for their own health, with confidence.

If you are one of these increasingly health- and prevention-conscious consumers, this book is for you. It's a book about health from the ground up, with the specific purpose of educating you about proper, preventive care of your most sturdy, yet abused and ignored, organs: your feet and legs.

But perhaps your needs at this point go beyond *preventive* care. Perhaps you picked up this book because you already have an annoying problem of which every painful step reminds you. Reading this book is a big step toward understanding your foot problem: what causes it; how you can prevent, mitigate, or reverse it; the benefits—and risks—of medical treatment; and questions worth asking your doctor.

More than ever, it is important to know how to properly treat and care for our feet and legs. With all the stress of living in cities and towns with concrete sidewalks, and working in buildings where pliable wooden floors have given way to much less resilient surfaces, we simply cannot afford to let our feet and legs take care of themselves. Until our feet and legs evolve to cope with the extra burden such hard surfaces (not to mention our penchant for fashionable shoes!) exert on them, it's up to us to cope *for* them. Educating ourselves about how our environment, our psychology, our habits, and our fashion choices affect the well-being of our lower limbs is the first step we can take toward easing the burden we place on them every day.

Much like our automobiles, our feet and legs have a way of letting us know when we have neglected to maintain them properly. They may let us know with little aches and pains that are the equivalent of our cars' squeaks and rattles; like our cars, they may immobilize us completely if we continue to ignore the messages they are trying to give us. We all know the truth of the rule Socrates expressed some twenty-five centuries ago: when our feet hurt, our bodies hurt, and as a result, our ability to function suffers. An intelligent, preventive approach can save us the time and effort it takes to treat and cure a foot or leg problem—not to mention the pain and inconvenience almost any such problem causes.

Such a preventive approach can begin in childhood, but it's never too late to start. This book is the first to outline *comprehensively* how anyone, of any age, can prevent foot and leg problems. It is geared toward parents who are concerned about helping their children put the "right foot forward" on a lifelong foot-and-leg-care program, as well as toward older folks who may have been plagued by foot problems most of their lives, and who may find themselves suffering from back or hip pain as a result. And it doesn't leave out anyone in between.

While all of us, at every age, can benefit from learning how to prevent these problems, at certain times we have special needs that require special precautions. This book also addresses those situations, highlighting in particular foot-and-leg-care programs for athletes, and those with illnesses that can affect the lower limbs—arthritis, gout, diabetes, arteriosclerosis, and psoriasis and other skin problems. And for those of us without special needs—those who simply suffer from occasional bunions, corns, calluses, athlete's foot, shingles, spurs, sprains, and strains, or who have suffered all our lives from flat or overarched feet—it will discuss the best at-home, over-the-counter, and professional remedies.

As concerned and caring as most health professionals are, they simply don't have time to explain everything they want to in as much detail as they would like to their patients. For foot and leg care, this book fills that gap. By reading it, you are giving yourself a "feet-first" approach to overall good health.

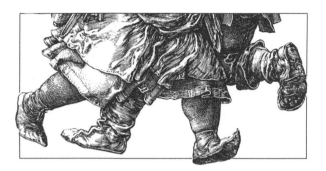

# THE
# NORMAL
# FOOT
# A Guide

1

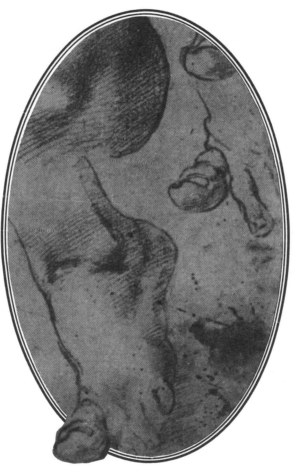

AWARENESS OF HOW you ordinarily look and feel—the "normal" state of your body—enables you to see the slow, insidious changes that precurse an *ab*normal condition. Here we will examine what a "normal" foot is and help you become acquainted with your own feet, so that you can detect any abnormalities as they arise.

## BECOMING FAMILIAR WITH YOUR FEET

Let's start by looking at the foot's normal *shape*. Don't worry if your feet are "abnormal" according to some of these criteria, though, particularly if they've been that way all your life: what is "abnormal" for some may be perfectly normal for others.

First, take a look at the overall line of your foot. Does your foot appear to be twisted in or out, or is the general appearance straight? If you trace your foot on paper you may find it easier to see. Now, look at your toes. The first toe should be nearly straight, with the second, third, fourth, and fifth toes curving just slightly. Toes that overlap or underlap are "abnormal," but in some people this causes no problem. The shape of the normal foot is smooth, with no lumps or bumps along the sides, or on top of the toes. Is your heel well-rounded and smooth, without bumps? Are your arch and instep high or low? If you notice that your arch is dropping, you know that something is changing, and you should have it checked. If you have smooth heels now but later see a bump developing on one of them, you know that something un-usual has happened. If you know what the "normal" shape of your foot is now, you'll be alert early to changes—for exam-ple, if the bones are moving out of position because of a structural imbalance.

And what about the size of your feet? We normally judge the size of our feet by our shoe size, but we may be wearing the wrong size shoes! It's not a bad idea to have your shoe size measured by a professional. Is the size of your foot in rough proportion to the size of your body? if it isn't—for example, if you are big and tall and have very small feet—learning what footgear is right for you now may save you trouble in the future.

Learn what your "normal" skin looks and feels like. Is it soft and supple, and evenly colored? Skin color should be uniform, with no red marks on the tops of the toes (in the joint areas) or anywhere else. What is its texture? Do you normally have hair on your toes, or not? A minute detail like the hair on your toes could alert you to a circulation problem if that hair starts disappearing. If you see that the skin on your feet is dry, cracked, or brittle, preventive measures *now* could protect you from ulcers and other skin irritations later.

In a full-length mirror, watch yourself walk. What is your "normal" posture? Is your head erect, are your shoulders straight? If your head and shoulders are slumped or dipped too far forward, or held back too rigidly, the rest of your body will be thrown out of line. Your chest should be slightly out, stomach slightly in. Look at the upper body as a unit. It should be held squarely over the pelvis, which should be in line with your legs, neither too far out, nor too far back. Do you throw your hips or your upper body forward when you walk? Too much of a forward thrust in either place can create an imbal-ance, which in turn can cause back, hip, knee, ankle, heel, or foot problems. Your arms should swing lightly from side to side.

Look at your feet as you walk. Each foot should strike the

ground on the heel, just slightly to the heel's outside, then twist slightly in. At that point, the foot should start to twist up again until "toe-off" occurs. This may sound complicated, but if you walk slowly and mindfully for a minute or so, you will be able to determine whether it is *your* normal pattern.

You can heighten your awareness further by observing what is normal for other people, and how you differ. Looking at pictures can help, too. If you now believe that you have posture problems that affect your walking, do yourself a favor: see a professional to help you diagnose, correct, and control them. There are lots of noninvasive ways to correct structural problems: exercise, manipulative therapy, and the use of orthotic devices. Seeking professional treatment can help you return to or maintain your "normal" gait and posture, which can prevent foot and leg problems further down the line.

## THE EVOLUTION OF THE FOOT

Long ago we used our feet, along with our hands, to swing from trees. Our toenails were especially helpful for maintaining a strong grip on the bark of trees. When our feet weren't taking us through the treetops, they were taking us along the ground—with our hands doing the other half of the work. Through many generations our feet gradually adapted to carrying our weight alone, and to walking miles across soft, grassy earth.

Interestingly, our feet have still not fully adapted to bearing our entire body weight themselves, and they are far from adapted to walking on hard surfaces like concrete. So they are still evolving. They are growing longer and wider, in response to the hard surfaces we pound them on. The bigger the area of the foot, the more the stress of the weight of our bodies and the pressure of the concrete is dispersed, and the less trauma there is to the foot as a whole. This evolutionary change is happening fairly rapidly: each new generation has feet larger than those of their parents. You can even see the change reflected in the sample shoe sizes displayed in stores: where the ladies' sample size used to be a five or six, it is now more likely to be a seven, or even an eight.

At the same time, our toenails are very gradually disappearing. We simply don't need them as we did when we were swinging from the branches of the trees. In fact, at this point they serve no purpose at all, and the same is true for our little toe. Scientists predict that in a mere ten thousand years our toenails and little toe will be things of the past. Over a longer period of time, our third and fourth toes will also disappear, leaving only our first and second toes, the only ones that we *really* use for walking anyway.

## PREVENTING PROBLEMS

In the meantime, because our feet have not completely evolved into organs for walking on hard surfaces, many problems develop merely out of the trauma that they take from hitting concrete. We have to take up the slack that remains between where our feet are from an evolutionary point of view, and what we *do* with them, which is something they are not quite ready for. In fact, every step we take on concrete is literally a shock to them.

How can we help them along? First, we must be aware that our feet aren't quite up to the treatment we give them, and second, until they are—which won't be in our own lifetime—we must provide the best possible conditions for them to take that treatment. We have to learn to baby our feet.

**SHOCK ABSORPTION**  A good start here is to invest in "shock absorbers" for your shoes—cushioned insoles. Or if you find yourself covering miles of concrete on a daily basis, go a step further and invest in a pair of athletic shoes—you can carry your dressier shoes along and change into them when you reach your destination. And walk on soft ground whenever possible. For those of us who live in cities, this may be impossible unless we make a determined effort to cultivate the habit of "taking our feet for a walk" in a park that has pathways made of dirt or grass. Walking is great exercise for your feet as well as the rest of your body, so this is not a bad habit under any circumstance. In Chapter 6 we'll talk about walking as an exercise program and give you guidelines about making it a challenge.

**MASSAGE**   A very pleasant way to baby your feet is to massage them. This is a good treatment for just about any foot problem, and everyone can take advantage of it. Two massage routines are described in Chapter 8; the first, which is easily self-administered, is a great way to start your day—it gives your feet and legs a head start on taking you where you have to go throughout the day, with as little stress as possible.

**EXERCISE**   Exercises specifically designed to keep your feet strong and pliable will give them an advantage. Walking is one of the best of these; there 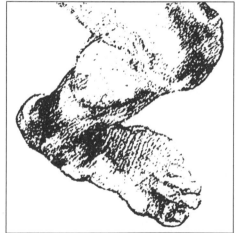 are also a few exercises you can easily do after your massage treatment. They take little time, but can make a big contribution to preventing the foot and leg problems that arise simply from living in the modern world.

This first exercise is great for strengthening the muscles in the fronts and sides of the legs—muscles that tend to weaken due to the powerful rear leg muscles that work against them. Imagine a six- to eight-foot-wide circle on the floor. Within that circle, walk a series of figure eights.

A good exercise to strengthen and increase flexibility in the toes is to try to pick up pencils or marbles from the floor with them. This is a particularly flexible exercise because it can be done any time you are sitting down—even if you are doing something else.

Another helpful exercise—and this one strengthens the toes, feet, *and* legs—is to draw the alphabet on the ground with the toes—and then again in the air—several times a day. Write each letter in capital letters or in script, or both.

## FEET FROM INFANCY TO OLD AGE

As we age, the needs and problems of our feet change. Here we will show you how to care properly for your children's feet from babyhood to young adulthood, and how to care properly for your own feet from adulthood to old age.

**INFANTS**   Be as familiar with your baby's feet as with your own. Don't let the responsibility for detecting problems lie with your pediatrician alone. You are the person who is in intimate daily contact with your baby, observing the changes in his or her body. If you see something unusual in the structure or positioning of your baby's feet, consult your pediatrician—or, better yet, take the baby to a podiatrist for expert advice.

In fact, it's really not a bad idea to take your baby to a podiatrist early in his or her life. Most podiatrists offer free screening examinations for babies, and often on a periodic basis (every two months or so), since babies' feet change so very quickly. That way, if there *is* a problem with your baby's feet, it will be detected—and hopefully corrected through relatively simple means—before it grows into a problem of major proportions.

Here are some guidelines for your own at-home observation of baby's feet. The first question is, as before, "What is normal?"

The whole rotated-out positioning of a baby's legs stems from the thigh bone's outward rotation. The rest of the leg and foot structure follows suit. Babies' feet are supposed to point outward—that's one reason Charlie Chaplin's walk was so endearing. Dr. Robins sees lots of worried parents who ask, "My baby's feet are all twisted out—how will he walk?" Out-toeing corrects itself, under normal conditions disappearing by the time the child is two. But in-toeing—pigeon-toedness—is *not* normal, and will not correct itself—though many pediatricians still leave it alone.

In-toeing is easy to define, and fairly easy to spot: when the toes point in toward each other, that's in-toeing. Diagnosing it in adults is particularly easy—check your footprints along a beach, or lay out a length of brown paper, powder your feet, and take a look at your trail. If you were to draw a line down the center of your trail on the beach, or down the center of the paper, your feet should point just slightly outward from that line. (Visualizing a clockface, if the line is at twelve o'clock, the right foot should point to one o'clock, and the left to eleven.) If they point outward, in-toeing is not a problem. In-toeing is a little harder to check for in a baby. If you notice that your baby's feet seem to turn in rather than out, ask your pediatrician to take a look. The younger your child is when you check for in-toeing the better, since it is best corrected at around six to eight months. It's easy enough to treat, depending on the cause, and usually doesn't involve anything as drastic or elaborate as putting the baby's legs in casts.

What are the causes of in-toeing? Sometimes it's a structural problem in the foot: the long bones may be twisted so that they curve inwards. Sometimes a muscular imbalance—easily corrected by exercise—is involved. But whatever the cause, don't leave the problem untreated. It is much easier to correct in infancy than later on.

What is normal in the baby's hips? Congenital hip dislocation, undiagnosed, can lead to foot and leg problems as well. An easy way to check for normal hip placement is to turn the baby over on its stomach, face down, and look at the creases behind the thighs. Do they line up evenly from side to side, or are they out of line with one another? If the creases seem to be significantly off, your baby's pediatrician should be alerted to the possibility of a problem. Another indication of the normal structure of your baby's hips is the "anchor sign" made by the two highest creases at the top of the thighs and the crack down the baby's buttocks in the center. Your baby's "anchor sign" should be well formed, with the line straight down the middle and the bottom forks evenly curved. Unevenness here, too, should be brought to a doctor's attention.

It is extremely important that hip dislocation be diagnosed and treated early; at that point it may be correctable by simple exercises that your doctor could give you, but later correction involves far more complicated and costly procedures. In the early stages of congenital hip dislocation, it can be treated best by casting. While I am not normally a proponent of casting children, as the long-term effects have never been studied, in this situation it may be necessary. When the problem is caught at birth, only a few months may be required. Bracing may be needed temporarily after casting, depending upon the doctor's experience and the patient's response to cast therapy. Each case must be evaluated by a competent pediatric orthopedic surgeon.

Always get a second opinion, but do it immediately. There must be no long delay in therapy. If the condition persists then surgery and casting for longer periods of time, as well as protracted therapy and bracing, may be needed. Obviously this adds up to a longer, more expensive and involved treatment, with no guarantee for success.

If you know what the skin on your baby's feet and legs normally looks and feels like, discoloration, inelasticity, or dryness will alert you to seek proper treatment at the right time. At the first sign of inelasticity or dryness you can treat your baby to a foot massage with oil. If the dryness hasn't cleared up in a day or two, you should have baby's doctor take a look.

What do your baby's toes look like? Toes that overlap or underlap could be considered normal, since many babies are born with one or both conditions, but should still be corrected early. You can do it yourself with a piece of tape or a small pad of 2 x 2 gauze, opened to its full length and then folded lengthwise. "Snake" the tape or gauze through baby's toes by lifting underlapped toes and putting the gauze under them, and depressing overlapped toes and placing it over them. When you finish, the baby's toes should be lying straight and flat. Consult your pediatrician or podiatrist as to how long to continue your baby's "toe-training" program, especially if you don't feel confident enough to embark upon this training program without professional advice in the first place.

Become familiar with your baby's toenails. Although nail infections and ingrown nails are fairly uncommon in babies, they can be effectively treated with simple "homestyle" remedies if they do happen. If you notice some redness around one of baby's nails, you can wrap the toe in gauze that has been soaked with Herbal Solution #1 (see Appendix B), or just plain warm water that has been brought to the boiling point. Allow the gauze to dry completely, and repeat. This old-time remedy acts as a poultice: the evaporation of the liquid draws out the inflammation.

It is as necessary to know what good hygiene is for babies' feet as it is to know what is normal about them. Proper footwear is part of good hygiene. One reason that nail infections and ingrown nails are not common for babies is that they don't wear shoes. Since babies don't walk, shoes are unnecessary—in fact, chances are that if your baby develops a toenail problem, it's because he or she has been wearing the wrong kind of footgear. If you want to keep your baby's feet warm, use socks or booties. Be sure that they aren't too tight; not only can that squeeze cause toenail inflammation, it can also push the toes out of position.

Proper foot hygiene also includes washing and massaging baby's feet, as well as clipping the toenails on a regular basis. It may surprise you to hear that no soaps should be used on your baby's feet and legs, unless they are dirty. Otherwise, only warm water on a daily basis is necessary, since your baby is hardly likely to get dirty enough to need a soap bath, which dries the skin. In the bath, make sure to clean between the toes, as well as washing baby's feet. Make just as sure to dry there, patting gently over the whole foot, rather than rubbing vigorously.

Babies love massage, and their feet and legs can especially benefit from it. After drying the baby's feet and legs, gently rub in a little sunflower, safflower, or soy oil, using the same technique you might use on your own feet and legs after a bath (see Chapter 8 for more detail). This is especially important for black or dark-skinned babies, whose skin tends to be drier than that of Caucasian babies.

Clipping the baby's toenails on a regular and frequent basis—once or twice a week—is part of a good hygiene program as well. Invest in a good, tiny nail clipper that is especially made for infants. The trick in clipping baby's nails is to clip straight across, never digging in on the sides. If it's impossible to clip straight across because the baby's nails are curving, you should have the baby's doctor or podiatrist show you how to clip them without cutting the child, or causing an ingrown nail or infection.

As you care for your baby's feet and legs by bathing and massaging them, or when you are clipping its toenails, you might notice that the nerve responses there are uneven and unpredictable. Don't worry; the infant's nerve supply to the foot and leg is incomplete at birth. Babies can't put their feet where they want them, or control their movements. During the first months of life, the nervous system develops; the unusual reflexes that you observe will right themselves.

Babies' feet are particularly delicate parts of their young bodies. They are extremely malleable, which is a big advantage when it comes to correcting problems early, and just as big a disadvantage, in that they are susceptible to pressure that could mold their feet the wrong way. The first step toward helping your baby start through life on the right foot is to know what his or her feet look and feel like, so that you will notice unusual changes and can then seek professional advice. The second step is to avoid any situation in which undue pressure is exerted on your baby's feet: tight shoes, socks, or sheets. Finally, good foot hygiene will give your baby a head start toward healthy feet for a lifetime.

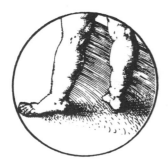

**TODDLERS** Once your baby starts to walk, it is as important as ever to observe his or her feet and legs. If you are in the habit of *knowing* your baby's body, and caring for it, the following guidelines will be a natural extension of what you are doing already.

By this time the outside edge of the child's foot should be almost straight.

If you notice that it is turning in, you should have your toddler's feet checked by his or her pediatrician or podiatrist, particularly if the outside of the foot has more of a "C" shape than a straight line. The bowed shape can mean metatarsus adductus—not an uncommon condition, but one that must be treated professionally.

A simple exercise can complement professional treatment for this condition. Sit in front of the child while it is lying on its back. Grasping baby's heel in one hand, place your thumb and index finger on each side of the foot, along the borders of the sole, so that the toes lie between your thumb and index finger. Then, very gently, place pressure on the outer side of the foot to straighten it. Hold the stretch for fifteen to twenty seconds. Remember, however, that the structure of your baby's foot is still highly adaptable; too much pressure can be harmful. This exercise, done five or six times in a row, twice a day, will help move the bone structure of the baby's foot back into the proper position, avoiding later problems. To supplement your at-home treatment, the baby's doctor may advise shoes that are padded to put pressure on the part of baby's foot that needs straightening. That way your baby can treat himself, simply by walking.

That endearing Charlie Chaplin–like out-toed effect should have disappeared by the time your toddler is two or so, when the thigh bones should have twisted enough so that the child's walk is relatively straightforward. If the foot and leg are still twisted out by the age of two, something is wrong. While out-toeing has been known to correct itself up to the age of twelve, it's better to get professional advice early while it can be corrected easily.

As your child begins to walk, it may seem to you that he or she has flat feet. This is no cause for concern, unless flat-footedness runs in your family. Your child's foot structure will be developing over the years, and that includes developing the arch that's right for his foot and body type. If flat-footedness *does* run in your family, then by all means have a professional look at your child's feet to determine what, if any, measures should be taken at this age to help the foot structure develop properly.

Something else that might concern you is that your toddler doesn't "toddle" as early as his friends do. Your child will walk when, and not until, the musculature in his feet and legs is ready to do the job. There is certainly no rush, and trying to make your baby walk before he or she is ready can cause undue damage to the muscle and nervous systems. Nationwide, the average age for the first step is sixteen months. This age varies, of course. In New York, for example, the average age is closer to twelve months. In other areas, to see a child start to walk at twenty or even twenty-four months old is not unusual.

Along the same lines, don't be alarmed if your child falls a lot when he or she is beginning to learn how to walk. To those of us who have been walking for some time, it all happens automatically, but to a toddler whose nervous system is still undeveloped and who is not accustomed to looking where he is putting his little feet, to fall is completely natural, and not symptomatic of any problem. Of course, if it seems that your child trips over his or her feet long after he should have learned the finer points of putting one in front of the other, you might consider bringing it up with a doctor.

Good foot hygiene for toddlers and small children is slightly more complicated than for infants, for the simple reason that they are walking. Therefore, their feet get dirty, and they need shoes. Soap becomes a necessity in bathing the feet. Massage is still helpful, with oil if your baby has dry skin.

Clipping the toenails is part of good foot hygiene at this age as well, although less frequently than when the child was younger. For most children, every three or four weeks is enough. Remember to clip straight across the nail.

Something new has now entered your child's world: shoes and socks. The most important thing to keep in mind about his shoes is that they be long enough. In fact, there needs to be at least half a thumbnail's length—that is, an eighth to a quarter of an inch—from the end of the child's longest toe to the end of the shoe. Call this "room to grow on," but make sure that it is there.

Toddler's shoes should be flexible. This rules out shoes that have leather soles so thick that they don't respond to the movements of your child's foot—very often, just the type of shoe considered "best" by parents and shoe salesmen. If your child doesn't want to walk in his new pair of shoes, it may be that they are simply too rigid. The proper pair of shoes for your toddler actually bends with his foot so that he can move the ball of the foot to "toe off" properly. As for socks, cotton is preferable because it allows your toddler's foot to "breathe," and is less likely to irritate the skin than a synthetic.

Shoes and socks are important; even in the house, your toddler is likely to pick up a foreign body in his foot by going barefoot. Even a tiny hair in a carpet can penetrate the delicate skin of a child's foot, causing pain, redness, and infection, just like a piece of glass would. The body may react to this foreign body by encapsulating it with a tumor, in which case minor surgery may be required to remove both the tumor *and* the hair, splinter, or whatever. Make sure that your toddler's feet are protected. In the house, socks or slippers are probably enough.

**OLDER CHILDREN**   Children between eight and twelve are much more active than younger ones, so, in a way, there's more to look for—and the signals you get can be confusing. There are *so* many changes happening that you'll have to draw on your knowledge of the child since babyhood to know what warrants professional attention.

You might notice that your child is knock-kneed, or just the opposite—bowlegged. The same child can appear one way one year, and the other way the next! Both conditions can and do occur within our framework of "normal," but if your child seems to be hampered in movement because of the structure of his or her legs, a doctor might prescribe a device to be worn inside the shoe, or simple exercises to stretch tight or over-developing muscles and strengthen others that are weak and underdeveloped.

Keep an eye on the skin of your child's feet and legs. If it becomes dry, give an oil or skin-cream massage for a night or two after the bath, and if the condition doesn't improve, see a doctor. The toes should be lying straight. There shouldn't be any new bends, twists, or swellings in the foot region. And by now the arch should be fully developed. In other words, you should be familiar with what is "normal" for your child's feet at this age, and therefore able to make a reasonably sound judgement about whether any change that does occur is worthy of a professional's consultation.

Daily bathing is still important to your child's feet. If your child doesn't go barefoot, soap is not essential; but if your child does, soap and a good daily scrubbing might be necessary for optimal care. By this time, washing his or her feet should be the child's own responsibility. Invest in a good cotton cloth so that the feet can be gently but thoroughly cleaned on a daily basis. And teach the child to dry between the toes!

Clipping the toenails is an even less frequent operation now—once a month is usually adequate. A straight-across clip is still the idea, although now that the toes are more developed, the corners of the nails may have begun to curve inward. If that's the case, the corners can be clipped in a slight curve, but never dig in deep.

Going barefoot results in one of the biggest foot problems for children; picking up foreign bodies which penetrate the foot. It's best (though almost impossible) to discourage going barefoot at all, and save yourself and your child a trip to the doctor, or worse, the emergency room.

And what about shoes at this age? Because the older child is very active, a running shoe is highly recommended. But there's a twist: if your child is involved in many different sports, you would be wise to invest in basketball or baseball shoes, or even a general-purpose sneaker, since running shoes are made mainly for unidirectional activity: i.e., walking or running. For the very active child, a shoe without the wide-flared heel of the running shoe may be your best insurance against future knee, hip, and ankle problems. In any case, most children this age have very little use for a leather-soled dress shoe. They need adequate support, easy movement, and protection, found in a lightweight canvas or nylon shoe.

**TEENAGERS**  By the age of thirteen, few children are going to want or need your constant observation of their bodies—in particular, their feet. In spite of the many changes going on in your teenager's feet and legs (they're getting bigger and bigger, if nothing else), by now he or she should have learned what is "normal" and what is not.

Your child should know what his or her feet and legs look like, be able to discern any unusual changes in their structure or skin, and know to call any reddened areas, irritations, blisters, black spots in the nails or skin, to your attention.

By the same token, your teenager can now take full responsibility for the hygiene of his or her feet. A thorough cleaning weekly may be enough, unless he or she is heavily involved in athletics. Drying between the toes is especially important. Biweekly or monthly toenail clipping should be part of the hygiene agenda, as well as massaging and moisturizing the feet on a regular basis.

At this age, foot massage assumes a new importance. A teenager's body is getting bigger, and the feet and legs are having to bear much more stress. Athletics may already be taking their toll on the structure of his or her knees, legs, and feet. In spite of your warnings, your teenage girl may have started wearing fashionable high-heeled shoes, which are definitely going to cause more stress to her feet. The daily massage program we outline in Chapter 8 is not a bad habit to encourage your teenager to develop now.

Teenagers encounter enormous peer pressure to wear those fashionable shoes that can wreak havoc on the feet. At the same time, this is one of the most important stages of life in which *not* to give into that peer pressure, which translates into physical pressure on feet that are still developing as well as adjusting to the shock of suddenly having to accommodate and transport a rather large body. As at any otherage, the teenager should choose shoes for good fit and comfort, not for fashion. But because friends' opinions may weigh more heavily than reason, you, the parent, may have to act as policeman and protector of your child's feet by *insisting* on good-fitting, comfortable shoes. Teenagers may not appreciate your concern now, but they almost certainly will later.

**ADULTS**   It is important for you to care for your own feet as assiduously as you do for your children's. *Observation* is the key. Learn what is normal about your feet and legs; notice any deviations from that normal state. Consult your doctor if

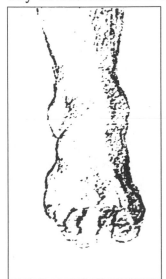

you feel that there is anything seriously amiss. *Maintenance* is the companion of observation. Maintenance of your feet and legs when you are an adult is even more important than it is to your children. As an adult, you have reached the peak of growth and are actually in a state of breakdown physically, little as we like to admit it. Maintenance here means good hygiene, regular exercise, regular massage, good nutrition—all on a daily basis.

Appropriate footgear for the adult foot is so important that we will be spending a great deal of time, in Chapter 7, discussing it. The same basic rules apply as in the other age groups we have talked about: good fit, good support, protection, and comfort.

**THE ELDERLY**   The same guidelines apply to the elderly, but more strongly. The adult foot is no longer growing, and is already beginning to break down structurally; the elderly foot is breaking down even further, a victim of the overall aging process.

If you are over sixty, observation and maintenance are more important than ever when it comes to your feet. The aging process subjects you to all sorts of conditions, such as arthritis, and most of them affect your feet simply because your circulation is not as good as it used to be. In addition, a change in your feet or legs when you are old may be a symptom of a much larger problem. For instance, swelling in the feet can point to general edema, which may be quite serious. Since your feet are at the tail end of the circulatory process, they can give you signals of what is happening in your system as no other organ can.

Good foot hygiene for the elderly is imperative. Bathing may not be as important as it once was, particularly since you may be more susceptible to dry skin. But moisturizing should be stepped up to twice a day, morning and night, using the same oils that we recommended earlier. You might want to massage your feet twice a day as well, when you moisturize, because it stimulates circulation in the foot and leg and into the joints. We recommend the Ten Minute Morning Massage (see Chapter 8) with oil or cream even before getting out of bed. It's a great way to start the day, and has a widely beneficial effect on the whole system. Stimulating the circulation in your feet and legs is a great insurance policy against the injuries to those parts that the elderly are so prone to.

# THE SKIN OF THE FOOT AND LEG

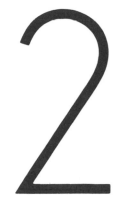

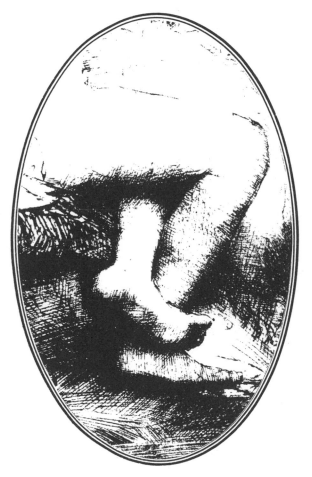

MANY DIFFERENT CONDITIONS can affect the skin on your feet and legs; this chapter discusses some of the more common ones.

## FUNGUS INFECTIONS

Athlete's foot, the most common fungus infection of the foot, usually develops as a result of excessive perspiration, and the ensuing sensitivity to a fungus that is actually *always* present on the skin. You cannot pick up athlete's foot from the locker-room floor, or infect others with your own case. Athlete's foot fungus grows on everyone's feet, and you can't catch what you already have!

If everyone has this fungus on their feet, why does it irritate the skin of some people and not others?

The skin of our feet is the habitat for thousands of microscopic creatures—a veritable zoo. Like any other environment, the ecosystem of this one is delicately balanced. Under normal conditions, the microscopic beings such as fungus and bacteria that grow on our feet compete with each other for space and food—some of them even eat each other—so that all are kept under control. But in excess warmth and moisture, or a particular chemical composition of sweat and tissue proteins, the fungus burgeons out of control. This ecosystematic imbalance results in athlete's foot; sensitivity to the fungus can assume the proportions of an allergy.

27

Athletes, as well as the rest of us, are prone to this problem when they repeatedly forget to dry their feet carefully, putting socks and shoes on while the feet are still damp. Simply through good hygiene—keeping our feet clean and dry—we can prevent fungus infections from growing. This is especially important for women who wear nylon stockings, which do not even absorb the excess moisture on undried, or ill-dried, feet.

The most common place for fungus infections to grow is between the toes. Along the bottoms of the feet and along the soles are other typical regions. Fungus infections almost never affect the top of the foot, other than up around the toes. While any skin condition that affects the top of the foot should be suspect, it is usually not a fungus infection.

A CHRONIC FUNGUS INFECTION looks like dry skin. You may notice that the skin is actually peeling. Sometimes it itches, sometimes it doesn't. It can form a line of demarcation along the sole of the foot, edging up the sides of the foot. The skin bordering this line may be dry, red, irritated, peeling, and cracked. In subacute fungus infections, there may be a breakout of little water blisters, and in the more acute fungus infections there are also breaks in the skin—fissures—that can become secondarily infected by bacteria. A fungus infection this acute is usually extremely itchy. It can also cause the foot to swell, which makes it painful to walk.

While fungus infections are not contagious to anyone else, they can spread on your own foot until the entire sole of the foot is covered, so all fungus infections—chronic, subacute, or acute—should be treated promptly.

For an ACUTE FUNGUS INFECTION, the best treatment is to wrap the foot lightly in a gauze bandage, elevate the foot and leg, and use a wet-dressing treatment with our Herbal Solution #1—an antifungal and antibacterial agent, as well as an astringent (see Appendix B). Pour the solution onto the gauze and let it dry completely. Then wet it again. This treatment should dry out the inflammation. Follow this procedure for twenty-four to forty-eight hours; if the acute stage has not subsided by then, you may need to consult a professional.

If what you have is a SUBACUTE FUNGUS INFECTION, or if your acute infection has been healed to that stage using the above treatment, you do not need the evaporative dressings. Instead, you should apply Herbal Salve #1 (see Appendix B) three or four times a day. Rub a small amount in until it disappears, wiping any excess salve away. It's what the skin absorbs that counts! If there are fissures in your skin, protect them by wrapping them lightly in a cotton gauze bandage. Keep your feet as cool and dry as possible during the salve treatment. The subacute stage should be resolved within three to five days.

The chronic fungus infection, one of the most common types, is also the hardest to treat. For one thing, people have a difficult time recognizing the dry skin along the border of the heel, the outside of the foot, and the tips of the toes as a fungus infection—so be suspicious of dry skin in these places, especially if it doesn't respond to treatment with skin cream or oil.

To heal a chronic fungus infection, use the herbal salve treatment three or four times a day. If in six to eight weeks the condition has not cleared away, you will need to seek professional care. Your podiatrist will more than likely prescribe a prescription fungicide such as chlortrimazole (Lotomin and Mycelex). A fungicide works its way into the skin and stays there, and is usually safe unless you have a reaction to the cream itself; but if your condition doesn't improve, or gets worse, it's time for another trip to the podiatrist.

While you are treating your fungus infection, it might also be helpful to apply powder to the skin on your feet. Do *not* apply the powder to the insides of your shoes, because the perspiration from your feet will cause it to cake and become a new medium for fungus to grow on.

It's always a good idea, but particularly when you have a fungus infection, to change your socks several times a day, if necessary. That's one of the best ways to keep your feet dry. Take a few extra pairs of socks with you to work and put on a new one every time you feel your feet getting sweaty. Cotton is best.

You can also use vitamins and minerals to help heal your fungus infection. A good program for that includes 1200 international units (IU) of vitamin E, 10,000 IU each of vitamins A and D, 50 milligrams of chelated zinc, and 5000 to 10,000 milligrams of vitamin C, all taken orally. (These quantities are for adults—they would need to be adjusted according to age and weight for children.) If you've ever had a chronic, subacute, or acute fungus infection, taking vitamins and minerals daily is as good a preventive measure as any.

**FUNGUS NAILS**   Nails, too, are part of the skin, and can suffer a fungus reaction which causes them to blacken, thicken, or yellow. The whole nail may rot, so it can be lifted right off the toe. There is no lotion, salve, drops, or any other outside chemical means that can help this condition.

One treatment that *can* help, however, is vitamin therapy. Vitamin E taken orally and applied topically to the skin around the nails, as well as vitamins A and D used in the same way, can improve the quality of your nails. Never apply the vitamins directly to the nails themselves. Rub them lightly all around the nail on the skin, and wipe off the excess. This treatment will improve the quality of your nails, whether you suffer from fungus toenails or not.

The only nonsurgical way to get rid of fungus nails, however, is through oral medication—griseofulvin, a prescription drug taken twice daily. But it usually takes at least three months, and sometimes several years, to eradicate the fungus through medication—and since there is a sensitivity (or even allergy) to the fungus already, it can recur, and you may have to go through the cycle of medication over and over again. The medicine also produces side effects that may have to be monitored through monthly blood tests. Just controlling the fungus by keeping your nails filed thinly with an emery board seems just as effective, with much less potential risk involved than taking medication.

If you're troubled by fungus nails, be aware that your condition can be worsened (or even caused) by water trapped under nails that have been softened by a long bath. Nail polish on softened nails will trap the fungus underneath the nail.

There is also a genetic sensitivity to the fungus—so your fungus nail problem could even be inherited.

As a last result, you could have your fungus toenails surgically removed—a painless process when expertly done. After the nail is removed, your doctor will recommend that you apply any one of a number of prescription fungicides (Fungoid Tincture or Synergine, for example) to speed the healing process. While surgery is often effective in curtailing a fungus problem, it is not without its risks, from bacterial infection to deformed nails that simply will not regrow. Surgical lasers have also been used to remove fungus nails, but the success rate is inconclusive.

## PSORIASIS

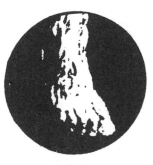

Psoriasis is a very common skin condition that affects the feet and lower legs. It can also affect the soles of the feet, particularly around the heels and other pressure areas, like the balls of the feet. Psoriasis is not a disease, but a condition—our body's way of ridding itself of negative energy such as tension, anxiety, and problems at work or home. With some people, stress manifests itself as stomach ulcers; with others, as psoriasis.

The symptoms of psoriasis are patches of reddened, irritated skin, with white scales. If you scratch one of these patches, it will bleed. The best treatment here is Herbal Salve #1 (see Appendix B) four times a day, particularly if your case is mild to moderate. For more severe cases, where there is a lot of thickening on the soles of the feet, it's necessary to rub the herbal salve into the feet at night, covering the feet with a plastic bag to help hold the salve's moisture in all night long. This helps the dead skin to soften, and in the morning you can just peel it off. A pumice stone may be helpful to gently scrape off some of the thickened skin.

While you're using the salve treatment, it's a good idea to cushion the tissue on the bottoms of your feet by wearing shock-absorbing insoles in your shoes, or even flexible, protective athletic shoes, to keep pressure off the affected area while it is healing. Another good idea is to wear cotton socks. Wearing cotton protects the healing tissue from the irritants in man-made materials (synthetics), particularly harsh chemicals. You should also avoid using soap on your feet—another potential irritant—as well as powders or other substances that might block up the pores in the skin and irritate the sensitive tissue further. Just wash your feet with warm water every day; then apply the herbal salve.

The best treatment for psoriasis is to recognize that you are taking your daily tension and problems out on yourself in this way—relax! As you learn to change your attitude toward your problems, you may well notice an improvement in your psoriasis. Avoid using cortisone cream, which controls psoriasis very poorly, and ultraviolet radiation, which can further dry out and damage the skin.

Psoriasis, among many other medical conditions, can also affect toenails. The symptoms of any of these problems are very similar to fungus nails: thickening, yellow, ugly toenails. The same treatments are also applicable: keep your nails cut straight across and filed thin with a nonmetal emery board or nail file, and seek professional care if you deem it necessary.

Bloody toenails, which look very similar to fungus nails or those caused by psoriasis, are in fact the result of the toe jamming against the front of the shoe and bleeding under the nail. They are more a sports injury than a skin disorder, and as such are treated in Chapter 5.

## WARTS

It is quite common to get warts on the bottoms of the feet, called plantar warts. Any wart is a virus that gets innoculated into your system through a break—even a tiny one—in your skin. You can pick it up simply by walking around barefoot after a shower, or getting out of a swimming pool to a sea of wet concrete, when skin has been softened by the water.

Once the virus enters your system, it secretes an enzyme that prevents your immunological system from detecting the virus. Therefore, no antibodies are produced as a defense.

The body is smart enough to use its second line of defense, surrounding the virus with a tumor of skin cells to prevent it from spreading, but that second line of defense sometimes just isn't good enough—the "mother" wart virus cell will send out "daughter" cells, like a bunch of grapes, and the virus will spread.

Under a microscope, a wart looks very much like a head of cauliflower, with nutrient arteries as stalks, bringing nutrients to the surface. When a wart is cut across the top, little pinpoint dots of blood appear: a diagnostic sign that a wart exists. Another sign is that skin lines do not go through a wart, ending at the very edges of the wart itself; when the wart is gone, the skin lines will reappear.

Eighty percent of warts disappear by themselves within two years. Why? Warts have a curious psychological component. Once your body understands that there is a wart in a certain area, you can actually "think" it into an antibody response which will eventually kill off the wart. This can be done with several different means, particularly with children: painting on "magic water"; buying the warts off for a quarter each; having the child draw a circle that represents the wart and erasing it a piece at a time each day. All these methods have helped cure warts. But if a wart has existed for at least two years, then it should be treated with other means, particularly if it is in an area that can cause discomfort (such as a pressure point like the heel). There is always the possibility that the wart virus will spread, or that the wart will become larger, causing problems in treatment later on.

In trying to eradicate a wart, it is important not to use over-the-counter remedies, as most of these remedies contain an acid which dissolves the wart—and can dissolve the skin around it as well! Professionals may heal warts with acid, but they use it very carefully to cause a skin irritation that activates antibodies to come in and kill the wart virus completely. Other warts on the body will actually disappear at the same time the "main" wart is treated with this method.

An innovation in the professional treatment of warts straight out of the sci-fi movies is the surgical laser. This method, while often very effective, does have several drawbacks: there is no guarantee that the wart will not return, the cost is much higher than for more conservative treatments, and there is an added risk of destruction of the growing cell layer in the skin, which could result in the formation of scar tissue.

Other methods that professionals employ are electrodessication (use of an electric needle), liquid nitrogen or other chemicals that cause blistering, and the surgical removal of the wart itself. All these methods have a high recurrence rate, because of the wart virus's ability to spread by replicating itself. Furthermore, if the wart virus is located in a pressure area, the scarring which some of these methods—surgical excision and electrodessication, for example—can cause could be far worse than the wart itself.

## CALLUSES

Calluses—a thickening of skin on the bottoms of the feet, usually in a pressure area like the heel or the ball of the foot—are never "normal," except for people who walk barefoot on hard surfaces. Calluses, like corns, are a warning sign that should never be ignored.

If you have a normal foot structure, the fat pad that is under your foot should prevent callus formation by acting as a shock absorber. But if the bone structure of your foot is moved out of position, then more pressure is placed on "dropped" metatarsal heads, causing calluses to form across, for example, the balls of your feet. (Dropped metatarsal bones are those which have had their normal position lowered toward the ground; this often creates the appearance of a high arch when the foot is suspended in the air.) If your heel strikes the ground at an improper angle because there's a problem with the structure of one of your leg bones, or if you just happen to be heavy, calluses can also form.

Calluses are easy to treat at home by taking a warm-to-hot foot bath every night (don't use soap, which dries the skin). When you're finished, use a pumice stone or emery board to gently scrape the skin smoother; avoid metal implements, which can cut the skin. Then, rub oil into your skin—safflower, soy, or sunflower (cold-pressed oil is best, since its vitamins have not been destroyed)—until you can *see* that the oil is absorbed. Wipe off the excess. You might also invest in shock-absorbing insoles for your shoes, which will reduce the pressure on your foot, and might help the problem, if it is due to improper positioning. Lower-heeled shoes will take some of the pressure off calluses on the balls of your feet, while wider-heeled shoes can help, especially if the callus is on your heel, by dispersing weight as you walk.

If none of these methods decrease the calluses on your feet, seek professional care. If your bone structure is greatly out of position, a podiatrist can make an orthotic device to control your foot structure. He or she may even cover the device with a professional shock-absorbing material that can effectively reduce the pressure on your feet.

## CORNS

"Corn" is such an innocuous name for those hard, round, yellow lumps that sometimes grow on people's feet: it suggests that the corns that sprout on one's feet are as harmless as the grain that grows in the Midwest—a natural phenomenon of little concern. But corns are a symptom of a problem which, unless solved, can develop into a big crop of pain, not to mention medical bills.

Corns—small, usually round areas that may form either on the tops of your toes, at the tips of your toes, on the sides of your feet where the bunion joint is located, or even *inside* calluses underneath your feet—are a symptom of intermittent rubbing. They might be caused by extraextensions of bone—calcium deposits—pressing on your skin from the inside of your shoe, or the ground pressing on your skin from the outside. They can even be traced to a bedsheet tucked too tightly; indeed, patients in nursing homes often develop corns and calluses from that very pressure. Whatever the cause of the rubbing and pressure, the delicate skin on your feet can't take too much of it. It protects itself by thickening, growing a hard lump at the point of pressure. And there's your corn.

If the corn grows too large, and the source of pressure has not been relieved, it becomes part of the problem rather than the skin's protective solution, adding to the pressure against the skin and bone and causing even more pain.

The simplest treatment for corns is to reduce the pressure from the outside. You can do this by wrapping lambswool around high-pressure areas or using shock-absorbing insoles in your shoes. You can even glue extra little pieces of these shock absorbers underneath the areas you want to give extra protection. You can work on your corns by pumicing them down after a good long bath. Corn removers—available over-the-counter—are *not* recommended for the same reason that wart-removing agents are a bad idea: they are basically acid in nature, and that acidity can lead to chemical burns and irritations.

You may want to get professional help, if corns are a big problem. Most of the time, the doctor will simply cut away the dead skin. If that doesn't work, as a last resort he or she might surgically remove the bumps from the bone in his office; hospitalization is rarely necessary.

Remember: if a corn or callus is painful, that means inflammation and soreness inside the foot, under the skin, and around and in the bone. In that case, our guidelines for treating bruises and sprains (see Chapter 5) might be helpful.

## CONTACT DERMATITIS

Contact dermatitis, another skin condition that often affects the feet, can be caused by something as simple as a chemical in your socks to which you are sensitive. Your skin reacts to the irritation, becoming red and inflamed. Little blisters may form, or the skin may crack into fissures, which invite secondary bacterial infections. This problem can occur on any part of your foot, top or bottom. If it happens, you must find out why!

Try to find and eliminate the source of the irritation. Wash your socks with warm water only, using no soaps or detergents, which contain alkali that can irritate the skin. White cotton socks will eliminate potentially irritating dyes and synthetic materials. (it is highly unlikely that you are allergic to cotton, but if you are one of those rare individuals, switch to wool.) Change your socks regularly, particularly if you sweat a lot; perspiration can seep through your sock into the shoe and pick up irritating chemicals, which then circulate back through the sock to your skin.

If your shoes are causing the problem, by all means throw them out or give them away and find others that are not irritating. Even the most "natural" of shoe leathers have been treated with tanning agents that can be irritating. The glue that holds the leather together can also be an irritant. For some people, hypoallergenic shoes—made without many of the chemicals known to irritate the feet—may be the only answer. They can be purchased in orthopedic shoe stores.

The treatment for acute allergic contact dermatitis is the same as for an acute fungus infection. While you are trying to determine the cause of your problem, try this: elevate the foot and leg, wrap it lightly in gauze, and start applying the evaporating wet dressings using Herbal Solution #1 (see Appendix B). After twenty-four to forty-eight hours of this treatment, the condition should have subsided to a subacute stage. If that is the case, discontinue the wet dressings and switch to the herbal salve treatment, applying it three or four times daily.

If you suffer from chronic contact dermatitis, you may, like many others, choose to ignore your condition. But it is much better for you and your feet if you make efforts to eliminate it. Try to determine the cause of the irritation, switch to white cotton socks, and in the meantime use the herbal salve three or four times a day. Avoid cortisone treatment if at all possible; not only does it weaken the skin in general, it also does not really cure the condition.

If you find that one symptom of the dermatitis is itching, you can get quick relief by rubbing the area with an ice cube for several minutes. Avoid using aspirin to reduce the irritation, or antihistamines to control the itching; the side effects of either far negate its benefits.

Once again, if none of these methods work to control your contact dermatitis, consult a professional. There may be a secondary bacterial infection involved, and only a professional will be able to diagnose it.

## IMPETIGO

Impetigo is one of the only truly infectious foot conditions. Usually found in children, it starts with a crack in the skin which leads to a bacterial infection, usually around or between the toes. In the acute stage, it should be treated by a professional, especially since it is contagious.

In the milder stages, or in recurrent cases of impetigo, you may want to try treating it at home first. Dress the foot lightly in gauze and use Herbal Solution #1 to draw out some of the infection and inflammation. The child should be kept off his feet as much as possible, with his leg elevated. If within twenty-four to forty-eight hours the condition is the same or worse, you should seek professional care. Your doctor will probably prescribe antibacterial salve, along with oral antibacterial medication to control the infection.

## TUMORS

Like the rest of your body, your feet can develop tumors. As cancer of the feet is very uncommon, these tumors are usually assumed to be benign, but that is no reason to ignore a lump anywhere in your foot. If you have a foot tumor, see a professional: it just isn't worth letting it go.

Your doctor can tell you if you have a little fatty tumor, or a connective tissue (fibroid) tumor, or a ganglionic cyst, or any of the many other benign skin lesions that can affect the foot. It may simply be an ingrown hair or foreign body that has somehow penetrated your foot. There are many different causes of lumps and bumps, few of which have to be surgically removed, unless, of course, they are causing discomfort. Surgery is required only when there is pain when you walk, or, rarely, when the nature of the tumor is in doubt and a biopsy is necessary.

If you have a tumor on your foot and it is slightly uncomfortable, you may relieve the discomfort by wearing more comfortable, flexible shoes (such as athletic shoes), using lambswool to relieve the pressure, or investing in shock-absorbing insoles. You should also switch to cotton socks, so as not to add insult to injury with potentially irritating synthetics.

Nevi, or beauty marks, can also appear on the feet. These can be premalignant, and should be checked out by a professional, especially if you notice a mark getting larger or smaller, thickening, or secreting fluid. These are all danger signs. Even the disappearance of a beauty mark is something to talk over with your doctor.

**MORTON'S NEUROMA**   Pressure on the ball of the foot can sometimes result in pinching of the intermetatarsal nerves, which run between the metatarsal bones. The pressure and resulting inflammation of the nerves will first create burning, pins-and-needles, or tingling sensations in the ball of the foot, running forward into the toes. When this condition is allowed to continue without relief for a long period—many months or years—the fat around the nerves can congeal into a benign tumor, which is then called a neuroma. Dr. T. G. Morton first described this disorder many years ago, giving it its name.

Morton's neuroma is best treated by not allowing the pressure to create a neuroma in the first place, relieving it with orthotic therapy, massage, and comfortable shoes. Once a neuroma has developed, it can be diagnosed through nerve electrical conduction studies called electromyography—it will not show up in x rays.

## DRY SKIN

Dry skin on the feet is very common, especially among older people, whose circulation is often poor. If your circulation is bad, that means a reduction in fat secretion by the feet's sweat glands, which in turn means dry skin. The decrease in blood flow to the skin's nerves also leads to dryness.

Dark-skinned people tend to have dry skin; if you are dark-skinned, avoid using any soap on your feet at all. If you *must* use soap, make it one of the super-fatted ones—soaps with added oils, and low in alkali. Among soaps of this type are the dry skin soaps made by Dove, Neutrogena, and Alpha Keri. A caveat: many so-called "natural" soaps are high in alkali, so always check the contents before you buy. Better yet, just use warm water without soap.

If dry skin is a problem, take the time after your bath to give your feet an oil rub, using soy, sunflower, or safflower oil. Let your skin have a minute or two to absorb the oil while you rub. Then wipe off the excess oil—it does your skin no good unless it is absorbed. If your skin is *really* dry, try Herbal Salve #1 (see Appendix B), two or three times a day. At the same time, make a point of avoiding irritating chemicals—even the chlorine in your local swimming pool. The twice-daily routine is especially important if your skin is parchment-like or brittle; skin that dry can break or crack, inviting fungus or bacterial infections, and even ulcers.

Besides the dry skin oil treatments, try increasing the effectiveness of the circulation to your feet by undertaking a cardiovascular exercise program such as the walking routine we suggest in Chapter 6. Vitamins—A and D, C, E, and chelated zinc—are helpful in controlling any skin inflammation or problem, such as chronic dry skin. Try the amounts we recommended earlier in this chapter.

## BLISTERS

Anybody who has ever been on a long hike in the wrong shoes knows all about blisters. In fact, most of us at one time or another—whether from tight shoes or an over-long walk—suffered an irritating pinch that turned into a blister. When the skin gets irritated enough, it becomes inflamed. To soothe the inflamed area, a natural healing fluid, lymph, flows into the tissue and causes the outer layers of skin to die. At the same time, the fluid puts pressure on the nerve, which causes pain.

The best treatment for blisters is prevention. Through good hygiene, proper exercise, and appropriate footgear, most blisters will never have a chance to develop.

But blisters that have already developed can best be treated at home by the following procedure. First *gently* wash the area with soap and water. Next, wipe the area liberally with rubbing alcohol. Clean an ordinary needle by allowing it to soak in alcohol for at least fifteen minutes. When the skin and blisters are prepared, remove the needle from the alcohol and use it to create an opening near an edge of the blister. Allow the fluid to drain by gently pressing the blister with a gauze pad. Apply Herbal Salve #1 over the entire blister liberally and cover with a sterile gauze pad. Never rub the salve into the blister. If the blister refills with fluid, repeat the process. Never use this method to treat large blisters caused by serious burns. If the blisters keep refilling, then use the procedure outlined for Herbal Solution #1.

## INGROWN TOENAILS

Ingrown toenails are another common problem, particularly among teenagers and young adults—oddly enough, because younger bodies generally fight and control infection so well that they might not even feel the pain of an ingrown nail. The infection tends to open and drain, simply from the pressure of their shoes as they walk, and before they know it there is a serious infection. If the ingrown portion of the nail is not removed, the problem will flare up again and again.

If you let an ingrown toenail go without treatment, by the time you finally, out of sheer pain, see a professional, the treatment may be extremely uncomfortable because the nerves are so sensitive. It may even require local anesthesia for the nail to be removed. On the other hand, if treatment is sought early, surgery on the nail will probably be virtually painless. So it is important to seek professional care as soon as you realize that you have an ingrown nail, especially if you are in a high-risk category such as people with diabetes or poor circulation.

Surgical lasers now offer an effective means of removing ingrown toenails and permanently preventing their recurrence. Many podiatrists see this method as surgical overkill, unless you are allergic to the chemicals used in other, more conservative, methods, when laser surgery may be required.

## INSECT BITES

Insect bites, somehow, are especially irritating to the feet. Treat them as soon as you can by rubbing the area with ice, which prevents release of the histamines that cause swelling and itching. Rubbing the area for several minutes also prevents the toxins that were injected into you by the bite from spreading, because it slows down circulation. Repeat the ice treatment every ten or fifteen minutes, if necessary. Only if the bite was from an insect that might transmit disease, such as the tsetse fly, or from a poisonous spider, do you need to seek professional care. If it's a typical insect bite, ice followed by an evaporating wet dressing such as Herbal Solution #1 to draw out the inflammation is usually sufficient treatment.

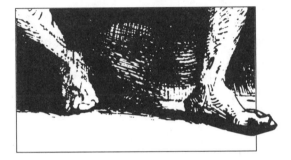

# THE CIRCULATION OF THE FOOT AND LEG

# 3

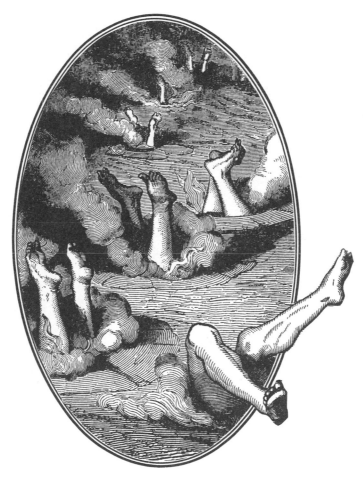

CIRCULATION IS, IN a sense, the ground of everything else we've talked about. Remember, your circulatory system holds the key to life for your entire body. It feeds your bones, your arteries, your muscles—every cell in your body, for that matter—with blood. If there isn't enough blood, your tissues will not get enough oxygen and nutrients to keep them healthy. And since the feet are most distant from the heart, at the tail end of the circulatory system, weak circulation will often show up in problems there first.

In this chapter we will treat problems with the circulation in the arteries, capillaries, and veins of the foot and leg. An awareness of the physiology of these vessels, as discussed in Appendix A, will help you to understand the causes and nature of these diseases.

## PREVENTING AND DETECTING POOR CIRCULATION

Regular aerobic exercise can prevent both arterial and venous disease from getting a "foothold" in your system. Because muscular contractions assist both arteries and veins to keep a regular blood flow, you can build up health in your arteries and veins by using your muscles. By *not* exercising, you are contributing to the breakdown of arterial and venous circulation in your feet and legs. With age, the circulation to the feet and legs becomes less efficient. Therefore, the older you get, the more important it is to do some kind of exercise to help the circulation in your feet and legs.

Exercise is also especially important if you spend a lot of time sitting down. Sitting for long periods can cause a vasospasm, or closing off of blood vessels, diminishing circulation to the feet and legs. Getting up and walking around the room for thirty seconds or so every fifteen to twenty minutes will help break the vasospasm and restart normal circulation. Sitting can also cause lower back pain and discomfort by putting undue pressure on our lower back, where all the nerves for the foot and leg originate. Often lower back pains will radiate down into the feet and legs. Again, to avoid this, avoid sitting still for long periods of time, and avoid leaning forward in your chair, which puts tremendous pressure on your lower vertebrae.

The way you eat is also important. If your diet is heavy in fats and cholesterol, you are inviting fatty deposits to develop in the arteries that feed your feet and legs blood, for example. If you smoke, you are inviting problems. Nicotine is a *vasoconstrictor*: it causes the nerves to make blood vessels contract, effectively stopping the flow of blood. This effect can be very dramatic, as in Dr. Buerger's disease, discussed in this chapter.

Because the hair on your feet and toes is fed by tiny blood vessels, or *capillaries*, if the hair on your toes, tops of your feet, or your legs disappears you should suspect a circulatory problem. Loss of hair in the extremities is one of the very first signs. Loss of hair may also result from wearing too-tight stockings or socks, which cut off the circulation.

Another sign of a circulatory problem is any change at all in the nails. If your nails become thickened, develop lines, or become weak or brittle, your circulatory system may be at fault. Your skin may also betray a weak circulatory system by becoming dry and brittle. If you are familiar with your feet and legs as they *normally* are, any of these symptoms will tell you very quickly that something is wrong, perhaps in your circulatory system.

## DISORDERS OF THE ARTERIES

The arteries have an elastic quality. If that elasticity cannot be maintained, because the arteries are not getting enough oxygen or nutrients, they deteriorate. Such deterioration invites calcium deposits. The resulting, hardening of the arteries—*arteriosclerosis obliterans*—keeps the artery from expanding to allow the proper amount of blood to flow down into the feet and legs. With arteriosclerosis come all the ensuing problems of poor circulation: lack of blood flow into the feet and legs, breakdown of tissues, pains in the legs and feet, loss of mineral content from the bones, muscle spasms, and muscle cramps in the calves of the legs, day and night. A vicious circle has been created.

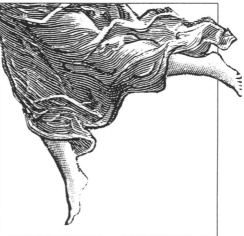

Spasms and cramps in the legs are a telling symptom of arteriosclerosis. Once this symptom is apparent in your sleep as well as when you're walking, the damage to the circulatory system can be pretty well documented by how many blocks you can walk before the cramps begin. Those "charley horses" that may plague your daily walk have a clinical name: claudication pains. Doctors call them 1–2–3–4–5 block intermittent claudication. The shorter the distance you can walk before the pain comes, the worse your arteriosclerosis is.

If you suffer from this symptom, you know that the only way to stop the pain is to stop walking. A rest allows your heart to pump enough blood into your feet and legs to wash away the waste products that have been building up in the muscle, which caused it to contract. Massage can help, too. However, one of the only ways to overcome arteriosclerosis obliterans itself is to exercise: exercising sends large amounts of blood into the feet and legs, forcing the arteries to open and close regularly, which keeps them elastic. You may have developed this condition by *not* exercising; exercising may reverse it.

You can also help by changing your diet. If you have been eating a heavy-cholesterol diet (lots of meat and dairy products, for example), fatty deposits in your arteries may be one cause of arteriosclerosis. Taking at least 1200 IU of lecithin daily is one of the best ways of nutritionally controlling fatty deposits, along with cutting down on the amount of fat in your meals. But again, one of the best ways of controlling the fat in your body is to exercise, because aerobic exercise—swimming, bicycle riding, walking, or running—uses fat as one of its main sources of energy. An exercise program such as the simple walking exercise program that we described earlier will also keep your circulatory system *moving*.

## DISORDERS OF THE CAPILLARIES

PERIPHERAL DIABETIC NEUROPATHY is a condition caused by poor circulation to the nerves of the feet and hands, due to a decrease in the fine microcirculation, or what is known as capillary circulation, in the hands and feet. This situation is brought on sooner in life by diabetes. When blood sugar levels are higher, this affects the peripheral nerves even more, sensitizing them. The only way to prevent diabetic neuropathy is to control the diabetes itself.

While diabetes is normally detected through blood tests, the symptoms of peripheral diabetic neuropathy may present themselves to the podiatrist. First, the patient may complain of excessive perspiration. However, that in itself is not enough to indicate the possibility of diabetes. We also have to look at other symptoms such as burning, pins-and-needles, tingling, itching, numbness and other unusual sensations to the feet which, along with excessive sweating, may be indicative of diabetes, prompting the podiatrist to suggest a glucose tolerance test or referral to a M.D. for further evaluation.

Keeping your blood sugar down to normal levels will minimize peripheral neuropathy, and regular exercise will maintain adequate vascular circulation throughout the body. Exercising aerobically is necessary, not anaerobic exercise.

In a severe case of diabetic neuropathy the skin may break down into abscesses and ulcers underneath the foot. This is caused by pressure on the skin from bones, as well as poor circulation to the skin. Diabetic neuropathy, since it deadens the nerves, will prevent the patient from feeling pain from these breakdowns until the ulcer actually forms. Severe infection usually occurs. Prevention of this starts with looking at the feet each day, moisturizing the skin and keeping them clean. This can prevent infection and make you aware that a breakdown is starting to occur.

Another problem that results from diabetic neuropathy is a drop foot. Once the nerves become numb, the muscles in the foot will actually stop contracting normally, causing the foot to flop down on each step. Again, the best way to help these problems is to exercise in a regular, aerobic way; keep your sugar levels under control; and wear proper protective footgear. Orthotic devices may also be necessary to control and stabilize the foot.

THROMBOANGITIS OBLITERANS—TAO—is another circulatory problem that affects the feet and legs. It is also known as Buerger's disease, after Dr. Buerger, who first described it in the early 1900s as a disease that primarily affected white Russian males who ate rye bread—the only common denominators that he found among the people he saw afflicted with TAO at Mount Sinai Hospital, New York City. After Dr. Buerger's time, however, some women also began to develop the disease. As it turns out TAO is not confined to rye-bread-eating Russian white males, but can strike anyone who smokes tobacco. Tobacco contains nicotine, which causes the nerves that control the blood vessels to misfire, thus closing the blood vessels down. When the blood vessels close down, circulatory problems develop. In fact, the circulation to the extremities—legs, arms, fingers, and toes—may be affected to the point at which gangrene and autoamputation take place. The frightening aspect of this condition is that, because nicotine affects different individuals in different ways, one person may have the same severe reaction from a mere puff on a cigarette as another person from a pack or more a day. Even more frightening, people with fingers and toes literally falling off will keep smoking, when the only way to stop this condition is to stop using tobacco in any form.

RAYNAUD'S PHENOMENON occurs more frequently in women than in men, being found in people who are deeply sensitive or emotional. Victims' nerves become so sensitized that they misfire, causing vasoconstriction just as in TAO. A lack of circulation to the extremities is the natural result. This phenomenon can also occur in people who are simply sensitive to the cold. Even in the summertime the most innocent warm breeze can cause a complete shut-down of the circulation to the fingers and toes in these highly sensitive individuals. (These are the people who complain of being cold when everyone else in the room is sweating. They *never* need air conditioning!)

Raynaud's phenomenon is more difficult to treat than the other circulatory diseases we have discussed so far. Treatment is not as simple as starting to exercise, changing eating habits, or quitting tobacco. So many habitual patterns are involved that those suffering from this condition need the most sophisticated psychological counseling. If you suffer from Raynaud's phenomena, you will need to learn to control your outflow of energy by learning to handle your problems in a more physiologically efficient way than simply shutting down your blood vessels.

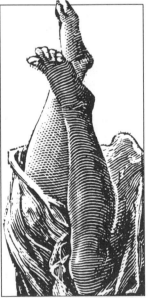

In the meantime, give your circulatory system a break by wearing proper shoes and socks in the winter to keep warm, and wear more than other people wear even in the summertime. You can also take the nutritional approach toward this condition. Take vitamin E in doses of about 800 IU three times a day, thirty minutes or so before you eat. (Vitamin E helps counteract Raynaud's phenomena by dilating your blood vessels, opening them wider, which gets more blood to flow to your feet and legs.) Niacin is also a vasodilator, and can help in the same way. At the same time, beef up your intake of Vitamin C, which strengthens the arterial walls, as well as the arteries themselves. Lecithin, as we mentioned earlier, keeps fatty buildups from occuring, which can also help. And once again, exercise can come into play here, helping you to increase your blood flow and opening up your arteries.

FROSTBITE results from a similar closing down of the capillaries. Not only those with Raynaud's phenomena are vulnerable to the cold, and it's not necessary to live in Alaska to get frostbite; in fact, the occasional freeze in warmer climates can be dangerous, as it takes people unaware. The blood vessels in the feet are very small, and those in the toes are the smallest in the entire body. When the foot is cold, it reacts by closing down these tiny blood vessels to conserve heat. If the blood vessels are closed down for too long, frostbite is the result.

Warning signs of frostbite are a painful burning sensation, followed by numbness. By the time your feet have gone numb, the circulation has been closed off completely for some time. You may notice that not only is the skin on your feet and ankles very cold, but it may be mottled purple and white. If you press on it, it may blanch even more, and the color may not return for a few seconds.

The first step when you've seen these warning signs is to rewarm the feet—slowly and gently—in lukewarm water, between ninety and one hundred degrees Fahrenheit. Circulation will return slowly, without a sudden painful surge, at this temperature. After about twenty or thirty minutes the tissue will be warmed up and relaxed enough for you to tell how much damage has been done to the skin.

If little damage has been done, applications of vitamins A, D, and E (in the form of an ointment) after rewarming the foot will be helpful. The skin should be protected with a layer of cotton or lambswool, and kept warm—warm socks and a warm room. More extensive damage—severely injured skin will turn black after a short time—and continued pain after rewarming require *immediate* attention at a hospital. Do not try to treat yourself. Delay in seeking professional attention may lead to loss of the toes from gangrene.

If you know that you have a problem with the cold, then try and protect yourself before you go out. Protect the skin with vitamin A and D ointment, or some Vaseline in a thin, even layer all over your foot. Wear undersocks made of a combination of polypropylene, cotton, and wool, to wick perspiration away from the feet and keep them dry and comfortable. Over these you can wear a thicker, heavier athletic or thermal sock—preferably of wool or wool and polypropylene. An undersock and a thick sock is much preferable to several pairs of thick socks. An insulating insole—one made for shock absorption will work well too—can keep the cold from reaching your foot from the ground. Finally, be sure that your footgear is of good quality and will protect you—look for waterproof shoes or boots with thick rubber soles and, preferably, an insulating lining material like foam rubber or fur.

Keep moving when you're outdoors. The more you move, the more blood circulates through your feet and legs. It's when you stop moving that you're at risk. If you start to feel your toes hurt or go numb, head for a warm place and give them time to warm up. Don't keep pushing it: a few extra minutes could be very costly. And avoid cigarettes, coffee, or alcohol before going into the cold. Nicotine and caffeine both can cause a contraction of your blood vessels and diminish circulation in your feet and legs. Alcohol, on the other hand, will open up the blood vessels and allow heat to dissipate from your extremities more easily.

Damage from the cold doesn't just happen outside. Warm socks and electric blankets help if your house is cold at night; you are especially vulnerable when you are asleep, as you cannot feel warning signs like burning and numbness, and you are not moving to keep your circulation up.

## DISORDERS OF THE VEINS

VARICOSE VEINS result from improper opening and closure of the lock systems—the valves we mentioned earlier—inside the veins. Even worse, those valves may be staying partially or completely open, a condition called "incompetent valves." If your varicose veins are a result of incompetent valves, the condition is very hard to regulate or reverse, because once a valve becomes incompetent, it is nearly impossible to make it "competent" again.

But there are ways to help relieve varicose veins, mainly by doing what you can to keep your blood flow up, in spite of the fact that the veins can't do their job properly. Again, exercise on a daily basis is one of the keys to helping this condition. By exercising, you are helping the blood flow *up*, counteracting some of the problems due to the damaged valves. Another way to ease the problem of varicose veins is to sit with your feet and legs elevated—waist-level, or slightly higher—whenever you possibly can. By doing that, gravity can help the blood flow back up.

You can also wear support stockings. Many different kinds of support stockings are now available; we recommend that you buy your support stockings in a pharmacy or surgical supply store. They may be a bit more expensive than some commercial brands in a hosiery or department store, but you'll be paying for *quality*, and it's worth it. These stockings will have an even gradient of pressure, one that will flow from the toes all the way up your leg. Cheaper brands do not maintain an even gradient pressure, and can actually do your legs more harm than good if you end up having pockets of blood collecting in different places where the elastic in the stockings breaks down. Parke Davis, Kendall, and Bauer & Black are known for their high-quality support stockings; Parke Davis even makes a sheer support pantyhose that has proven just as efficient in helping women with varicose veins as standard support stockings. For pregnant women, or the overweight, Parke Davis also makes a pregnancy support pantyhose with an expandable belly. (See Appendix C for addresses.)

If you have a severe problem with varicose veins, you may want to investigate custom-made surgical support stockings. Two companies in this country, Jobst and Sigvaris, make them. A podiatrist must first take measurements from your toes up to your thigh and send the measurements to one of those companies. If you go this route, be sure to have your measurements taken when your feet and legs are not swollen. Support stockings act as an alarm that tells you when your feet and legs are swelling; if they're measured to fit a swollen leg in the first place, that alarm system won't work when you need it.

If you have varicose veins and can't afford support stockings, sometimes an Ace bandage will give you the support you need. Wrap a three- or four-inch Ace bandage around the leg where the varicosity is a problem; this may require wrapping your legs from the toes to the groin, if you have a severe problem.

PHLEBITIS is a common adjunct to varicose veins. When the blood doesn't flow up properly because of varicosities, it starts to clot—a perfectly normal mechanism for slow-flowing blood. If blood starts to clot in the varicose veins, phlebitis, or inflammation of the veins—a dangerous condition—is the result. Phlebitis can also be caused by illness, an infection in the blood system, or a direct blow to the afflicted area.

Phlebitis is dangerous because a blood clot may loosen and travel from the vein to the heart, causing a heart attack, or the brain, causing a stroke. While the outer manifestations of phlebitis are almost nil—you don't feel sick or have a fever— the condition requires great care. Rest is the best treatment. By rest, we mean total bedrest, for ten days to two weeks. If you are suffering from phlebitis, you should not be walking *at all*—not even to the bathroom. You should stay in bed, at home or in a hospital.

The phlebitic area or areas will be easy to discern, because they are usually hotter than any other part of the body. But hot and cold compresses are *not* effective in treating phlebitis or varicosity problems. A *warm* compress, however, might prove helpful. Just take a kitchen towel, soak it in warm water straight from the tap, wring it out, and place it on top of your *elevated* leg for five or ten minutes. This method is a gentle way to help dry out some of the inflammation in the vein, the skin, and the tissue, yet it is not hot enough to induce part of ablood clot to break off and start its dangerous journey through the rest of your body.

Another symptom of phlebitis is pain in the affected area. This pain—called Homans' sign—is especially noticeable in cases of acute deep thrombophlebitis—phlebitis with clotting of the blood. A side effect of phlebitis is that the skin on the legs may develop little dark spots, hemosiderin deposits. These spots result from a breakdown in the blood vessels of the affected areas. Hemosiderin—the pigment that makes our blood red—falls out of the blood, since it is heavier than the blood itself, goes through the blood vessel wall and tissues, and eventually becomes trapped in the deeper layers of our skin. Once these spots appear, they will not go away; the deposits are trapped permanently.

Another sign of phlebitis—or any varicosity at all, for that matter—is that the skin in the troubled places becomes dry, brittle, and itchy. It may even crack and peel. Itching is a sign of nerve damage from poor circulation, but one of the worst things you can do for this itch is to scratch it. The dry skin will react by breaking and bleeding; your body may not be able to heal this area efficiently, because the circulation there is already so poor, and the little break may become bigger and deeper until you have a bacterial infection that festers into an ulcer. The ulcer could be almost impossible to heal, taking weeks or months.

Any superficial break in the skin over a varicose area in your leg must be treated promptly to avoid an ulcer; Apply our Herbal Salve #1 (see Appendix B) to the spot three or four times a day, and then cover it with sterile gauze. If you notice that the slight break is becoming bigger, seek out professional help *before* it becomes a big problem.

If you have any circulation problems, swelling in your feet and legs might also be a problem. There are several ways to effectively reduce or relieve that swelling. Become aware of your daily intake of salt and cut it down as much as possible. You can also elevate your feet and legs whenever you are able, and avoid standing still—walking is one of the best treatments for a swelling problem. Good foot and leg hygiene are more important than ever if you have problems with your circulation. Your skin is not receiving the oxygen and nutrients it needs, and is therefore far more vulnerable than usual to bacterial infections. If you keep your feet and legs clean and keep your skin soft and supple by massaging it with oil every day, or twice daily if necessary, you are giving your feet and legs the best defense against ulceration and other forms of breakdown.

# THE JOINTS
# AND ARTHRITIC
# DISEASE

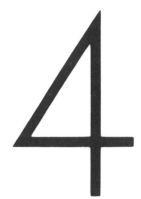

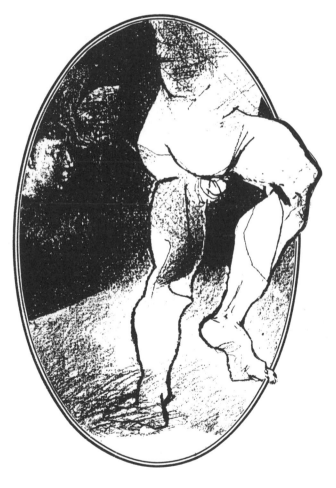

ARTHRITIS IS AS misunderstood as it is common (one in seven people in the United States suffer from some form of arthritis). The word summons up images of people crippled by pain, but this is not necessarily the case with many people who have arthritic problems. After years of investigations by thousands of researchers, resulting in hundreds of journal articles and dozens of books, we know little more today than we did half a century ago about the group of conditions called the collagen or arthritic diseases.

First, while arthritis affects the joints, the arthritic symptoms of joint pain and stiffness can also result from other conditions—accidental injury, over-exercise, or food allergies, to name a few. And, second, arthritis is not really only one disease. There are at least sixteen distinguishable forms of arthritis, with different causes, symptoms, and prognoses, affecting young as well as old and varying from a barely noticeable stiffness to a disease which can attack the skin, muscles, blood vessels, and eyes as well as destroying joints completely. Of the many kinds of arthritis three of the most common, which we will treat here as they often affect the foot and leg, are osteoarthritis, rheumatoid arthritis, and gouty arthritis.

## OSTEOARTHRITIS

Osteoarthritis is the most common form of arthritis, though its symptoms are often mild. In fact, almost everyone who lives a natural long lifespan probably develops some degree of osteoarthritis, although they may not even notice it in its mild 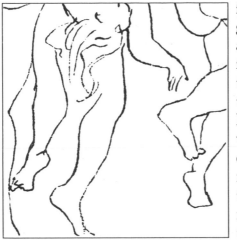 form. Osteoarthritis is a degenerative disease, most often affecting those over the age of forty-five. It primarily attacks the weight-bearing joints of the feet, legs, and lower spine. In these joints the cartilage which cushions the joints become softened; its fibers separate and disintegrate. The thinned cartilage results in irritation of the *perichondrium*, the tissue that covers the cartilage, and of the *periosteum*, the lining of the joint itself. This irritation stimulates bony growth—known as *bone spurs*—at and within the joint; eventually these can make joint movement difficult and painful.

Osteoarthritis that develops with no specific cause, over the years, is called primary osteoarthritis; sometimes trauma to a joint, such as a sports injury or an infection, can trigger what is known as secondary osteoarthritis. Although many believe that primary osteoarthritis is the inevitable result of wear and tear, researchers are investigating the possibility that an inherited weakness in the cartilage, a failure of the synovial fluid to lubricate properly, or a slight abnormality in the structure of the joint itself may sometimes be responsible. Not much can be done to prevent primary osteoarthritis; at the first signs that it is developing it is important to minimize stress to the affected joints. One way to do this is to lose weight, as obesity puts unnecessary pressure on weightbearing joints. Treatment of developed osteoarthritis involves pain control, improving and maintaining movement in the affected joints, and sometimes surgical correction. Aspirin reduces both pain and inflammation and has few side effects. Exercises to keep the joints from stiffening can be undertaken in water, to keep the weight off the joints. In severe cases a badly affected joint can be replaced entirely with an artificial one, a technique that has proved particularly effective with the hip and knee. Another surgical procedure involves removing pieces of bone or cartilage that might be irritating a joint.

## RHEUMATOID ARTHRITIS

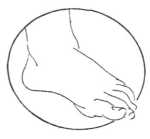

Rheumatoid arthritis is systemic; that is, it affects the connective tissue all over the body, not only in particular joints, and can also attack the skin, muscles, and blood vessels. An early sign of rheumatoid arthritis is an inflammation of the synovial membrane which lines the joints. In the second stage the synovial tissue thickens and is called a *pannas*, which grows inward along the cartilage surface, damaging it. A tough fibrous material, or *fibrous ankylosis* (ankylosis means immobility of a joint), develops and adheres to the joint, preventing its motion. In the final stage this fibrous material can ossify, developing into a *bony ankylosis*.

The causes of rheumatoid arthritis remain elusive, despite all the research that has been devoted to the subject. It is thought that it involves an over-reaction by our immune system; some researchers believe that an allergic reaction to certain foods may be a factor. This form of arthritis is best controlled by approaching the problem in several ways at the same time. It is much easier if you can do something *before* the condition has become crippling. Even then, however, it is never too late to work at improving your condition, and preventing it from worsening.

A change in diet is essential, with no cheating. All of the following foods must be absolutely eliminated: the belladonna family of vegetables (onion, tomato, pepper, eggplant); refined sugar in any form; refined starch; salt; milk and milk products; artificially colored foods; preservatives; yeast; citrus; meat; poultry; and any other food you feel you are sensitive or allergic to. These foods must be eliminated at once, not gradually over time. Next, place yourself on a four-day rotation plan; that is, avoid eating the same food on more than one day in each four-day unit. For example, have rice at each meal if you wish in one day, but not again for the next three days. As you introduce a new food into your diet each day, observe your body's reactions. Any increase in arthritic symptom, allergic reactions, or feeling of weakness or fatigue should warn you to eliminate that food. Those whose diet has been very toxic must sometimes go on a controlled fast for several weeks to eliminate the symptoms of this toxicity.

At the same time, supplements can be added to your diet. All the vitamins and trace minerals are needed, as well as large doses of vitamin C (as much as your intestines will allow without distress).

An aerobic exercise program will complement these nutritional changes. Swimming has proven best for arthritis sufferers; if you can't swim, walking in a pool is recommended, as the water reduces body weight, and thus, the pressure on joints. Exercising also stimulates the body to create several natural chemicals such as endorphins, which can help mitigate the pain of arthritis and bring about a general feeling of well-being. Exercise should be daily to effectively maintain the level of these chemicals as well as the flexibility of the joints. Avoid gravity sports such as running, though; these can damage already inflamed joints.

Diet and exercise are the easy parts of this arthritis treatment; the third part, spiritual awareness, is the hard one. Eliminate all your sore, painful, congested, unkind thoughts, whoever or whatever they may be about. Don't be frightened away by the implications of such a life change. Only in ridding yourself of negative thoughts and emotions can you hope to free yourself of the painful effects they have had on your body.

## GOUT

Gout is a metabolic disorder, but its major clinical sign is arthritis. It is most common in men over thirty to thirty-five years old. In people prone to gout the kidneys cannot cleanse the blood of excess purines, which are the end result of protein metabolism. Uric acid builds up in the blood, and is eventually deposited in the form of crystals in and around the joints. These joints become painful, reddened, hot, swollen, and exquisitely sensitive to the touch.

An attack of gout may be brought on by injury, cold, or stress. It can be diagnosed by an excessive level of uric acid in the blood approximately two weeks after an attack has ended; during the attack itself the uric acid is concentrated around the joints and blood levels are low or normal. Gout can be treated during an attack by colchicine, a medicine extracted from the bark of a tree. This will usually stop a gouty attack within hours, but has strong, though short-lived, side 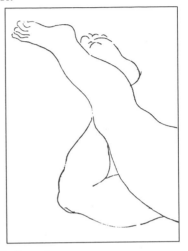 effects of gastrointestinal cramps and diarrhea.

It is important to control gout; recurrent attacks can affect the bones and joints of the feet permanently, causing them to be broken down and then rebuilt abnormally. Chronic pain and difficulties in walking can be the result. Most people don't need medicine to control their gout, however; the best way is through diet. The following foods, which are high in purines, should be completely avoided:

Beef, pork, and red meat of any kind
Organ meats—kidney, liver, brains, sweetbreads
Whole grains in any form
Shellfish, anchovies, sardines, herring
Alcohol
Coffee, tea, and other caffeinated beverages
Lentils and lima beans
Fried beans of any kind
Celery, radishes, mushrooms, peas, spinach, watercress, asparagus, cauliflower
The belladonna vegetables—onion, eggplant, tomato, pepper

Eliminating these foods reduces your chances of ever having a gout attack. People with gout often seem to fight this simple approach to prevention, but the alternative, long-term gout control medication, can have adverse side effects on your kidneys.

# SPORTS
# MEDICINE

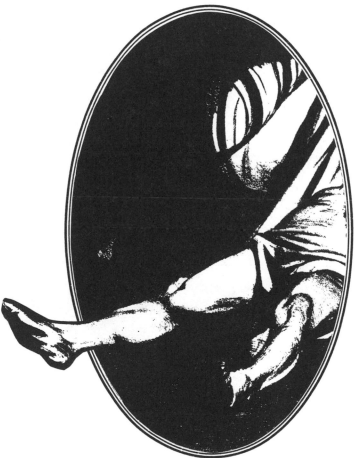

FOR ATHLETES IN any sport, the feet and legs are particularly vulnerable to injury. Here are some tips about foot and leg injuries that are common for athletes: how to prevent them, how to recognize them, and how to treat them when they do happen.

## TOENAILS

Toenail injuries are common in athletes who wear poorly fitting footgear. No matter what sport you play, play fair with your feet first by wearing shoes that fit. If your shoes are too tight, whether you run, jump, slide, dance, skid, or skate, your toenails will jam up against the end of your shoe, resulting in bleeding under the nail. When the blood dries, you have a black nail. If the skin and nail are badly damaged, the nail will even fall off. Although our bodies can manufacture new toenails, if they have to do it enough times through our own carelessness, they can't do it properly. If you traumatize your toes time and time again, the result will be deformed new nails—nails that are thicker than the old ones, dark colored or yellowish, with thick lines across them. Once these nails form, there's nothing you can do about it. There *is* something you can do now, though: make sure you buy the right shoes for your sport, and that there's at least a thumbnail's width between the tip of your longest toe and the end of the shoe.

If you have the right shoes, and they fit, and you're still plagued by black toenails your problem may be fungus related. A fungus toenail can look a lot like the black toenails caused by bleeding under the surface, but they are much harder to avoid, because they are the result of a sensitive reaction to fungus on the toes. Their treatment is discussed in Chapter 2.

## TOE JOINTS

Toe joint injuries plague athletes of every sort. These joints are very easy to jam: all you have to do is jump onto a toe that happens to be bent under your feet, or come down on your foot at the wrong angle. If the pressure is sudden enough, you will feel a sharp stabbing pain and hear a snapping sound in your toe.

What does that sound mean? Probably you've torn a ligament, the sinewy tissue that holds the bones of joints together. Or you might have injured a tendon, the tissue that connects the muscle to the bones. Trust that sharp pain you feel: even if the ligament or tendon is only partially torn, it will cause swelling, and can take six weeks or longer to heal. Especially because this kind of injury takes so long to heal, it's important for you to take the time at the beginning to help it along. *Stop playing* immediately, get off your foot, and elevate it. Apply an icepack to keep the swelling down. Do this off and on for a good twenty-four hours, then start moving the toes to prevent adhesions or scar tissue from forming. Remember to move your toes regularly, even though it may be painful—adhesions or scar tissue can inhibit future normal movement.

When you're ready to get back to your sport, tape the injured toe with half-inch paper tape. It's important not to tape it too tightly, or your circulation will be impeded. Just wrap it gently so that there is some compression. If it helps to tape it to a neighboring toe, do that as well. The point of taping your toe correctly is not simply to strengthen it a little, but also to give you a built-in alarm: if your toe starts to swell again, you can feel it, and get off your feet before you've injured yourself again. If the toe does start to swell during play, remember to elevate it.

But what if that "snap, crackle, and pop" that you heard was *not* a ligament or tendon tearing, but a bone breaking? How would you tell? A broken bone doesn't just swell, it also turns black and blue. Look for black-and-blue marks even further up the foot than where the suspected broken toe bone is: when a bone breaks, so do a lot of blood vessels. If you think you've broken a bone, get a professional to look at it, no matter how simple a matter it appears to be.

Pain is rarely so definite that it is certain to be immobilizing; in fact, sometimes when we must keep moving—propelled by stress, speed, or necessity—we choose to ignore pain, labeling it "annoyance" instead. Our body cooperates, producing chemicals that numb the pain at the site; our nerves cooperate by being so traumatized by the injury that they don't transmit the feeling of *pain*. All these factors can add up to ignoring the fact that we've broken a bone in the foot. Even if you can walk on it, get it checked out to prevent problems later. An improperly set toe might never function fully again.

## METATARSAL JOINTS

The metatarsal joints of the foot correspond to the knuckles of the hand. Because they are joints, they also have ligaments or tendons that are subject to tear with wear, and bones that will break. In sports like basketball, baseball, tennis, racquetball, dancing, and many of the martial arts, you can easily twist the bones in your foot after you've landed in a new place, or jump at an odd angle and land improperly on your feet, subjecting these joints to injury.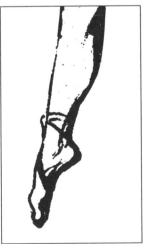

You'll know if you injure your metatarsal joints by the same symptoms as if you injure your toe joints: sharp, stabbing pain, perhaps a crackling snap, and swelling. If you've broken a bone, it will likely let you know by turning black and blue. Treatment, too, is similar: elevation, ice, and an Ace bandage or compression dressing immediately, as well as motion therapy after the first twenty-four to forty-eight hours to prevent adhesions or scar tissue from affecting your future mobility. Here, too, once you're back on your feet, taping can act as a "smoke alarm" for you to get *off* them if swelling occurs. In addition, taping can strengthen the injured area and keep swelling down. These injuries, too, take a good six weeks to heal.

A common metatarsal joint injury is popularly known as "judo joint," because judo afficionados are most likely to 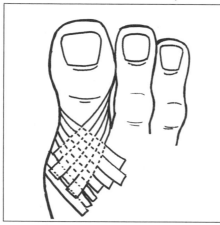 suffer it. Judo is practiced barefoot on a floor mat, and one move is to grab the mat with the big toe as the foot twists. The result is frequently injury of the first metatarsal joint (the one under the big toe). With this injury, basketweave strapping of the toes can be very helpful in preventing excess swelling, speeding the healing process, and alleviating pain. This technique (see picture) also allows a certain amount of joint motion even though the foot is taped.

The metatarsal joints are also subject to STRESS FRACTURE, a complete or partial break in a bone caused by its inability to tolerate repeated, rhythmic stress. That's different from the fracture caused by a sudden, intense force. How can you tell if you have a stress fracture? When you start working out, you feel pain. As you continue, the pain feels worse, but then when you're through, you feel little pain, or even no pain at all.

A stress fracture will usually heal by itself. All you have to do is decrease your workout to about half your normal time and intensity and give your feet a chance to rest. If you do that and the pain continues, stop your sport for at least two weeks. When you resume, start with about a quarter of your former time and intensity. Work up to your previous normal level very slowly, at the rate of perhaps only a ten percent increase in activity every two weeks. That way, your bone can heal completely, while regaining strength at the same time.

MARCH FRACTURES, so named because many World War I soldiers suffered them simply from marching too long and hard, can occur if you work out too heavily at the beginning of the season on bones that have been relatively idle, or if you overdo in a new sport. In either case, your bones are simply not strong enough to take the pressure you are putting on them. Your foot will hurt and swell, and may even turn black and blue. Here, the pain doesn't stop when you stop working out, the way it can with a stress fracture. See a professional; the bone must be set properly to prevent complications later. If you do that and avoid all athletic activity for at least eight weeks the fracture should be healed. But remember, as with a serious stress fracture, re-embark on an athletic program slowly and with care.

## ARCHES

In pursuing your sport, you might notice pain *under* your foot along the arch. Such pain is symptomatic of two common conditions: strain to the joints, ligaments, tendons, or muscles that run under the foot, or plantarfascitis.

The first condition—strain to one or more of the many components under the foot—is most likely to happen if you have high, rigid, arched feet. If you're flat-footed, you're unlikely to suffer such strain, but you could be suffering from plantarfascitis—inflammation of the plantarfascia, a sheet of fibrous muscle tissue running from the heelbone to the metatarsal bones, underneath the foot. The plantarfascia can be strained at any point from the heel to where the toes begin, and can trouble both athletes with flat feet and those with high arches.

Both these conditions require the same treatment: extra arch support. Athletes should tape the ailing foot: shoe inserts don't work nearly as well. Taping the foot for extra arch support is a temporary, but sometimes useful, way of relieving pain or strain to the arch. Strappings of tape have been used for many years in athletic injuries to reinforce support and to limit the motion of muscles, tendons, and ligaments. Unfortunately, the most recent studies have shown that within thirty minutes to an hour most of the benefit will be lost due to sweating, slippage, and stretching of the tape. However, for approximately the first twenty minutes in athletics, and for longer periods in people who limit their movement of the taped part, taping may have pain-reducing and reinjury-preventing qualities.

Using either flexible cloth adhesive tape or elastic adhesive tape (available in some pharmacies and most surgical supply stores) one-and-a-half to two inches wide, cut into eight-to-ten-inch long strips, the arch is reinforced in the following manner. Begin at the front of the heel where the arch starts. Place one edge of the tape about one-and-a-half inches up on the top of the outside of the foot just in front of the outside ankle bone. Pass the tape under the foot, pulling gently on the tape as you lay it against the skin. The tape should gently lift the arch of the foot up, to prevent it from flattening. The tape should end up on top of the inner side of the foot, just before the tendon which goes to the big toe (found there by lifting your big toe up towards your body, away from the ground). Never cover this tendon with tape as it will stop it from moving and could cause tendonitis. Overlap the first strip of the tape with another by approximately one-half inch and continue with additional strips of tape until the entire bottom of the foot in the arch area is covered by overlapped tape. It is important to protect the skin from the negative effects of prolonged strapping with tape by using a special solution, sold in surgical supply stores for this purpose. This can also prevent tearing of adhesive-weakened skin and reduce allergy or sensitivity to the tape adhesive.

People with poor circulation, such as diabetics and the elderly should not apply tape without professional advice on its safety and use.

If taping doesn't work, you might invest in one of the many over-the-counter orthotics available, such as Dr. Scholl's "runner's wedge." There are many such inserts on the market, most of which cost less than twenty dollars—inexpensive enough to experiment with. Just make sure the support is light and flexible—stay away from those made with steel.

If you've got a serious arch problem, the podiatrist, can make a specially fitted support for your foot. This is more expensive than an over-the-counter device, but well worth the money if nothing else seems to help.

## HEELS

Like the metatarsals, the heels are vulnerable to stress fractures when they're overused. The symptoms tend to be the same: pain that increases with exercise, and decreases when you stop for rest. The treatment, too, is identical: take some time out from your sport and give your heels a rest.

Heelspur syndrome, another common problem for athletes, is characterized by an "off-and-on" pain which is noticeable when you start to play, then decreases, then flares up again with continued play. If you stop to rest, you'll notice a decrease in the pain, especially if you elevate your foot. But as soon as you try to walk on it, the heel hurts so much that you might find yourself limping. Oddly enough, if you persist and keep walking, the pain again recedes. This condition, untreated, will only get worse. At first, you may be able to continue to play your sport, but over time the pain will become so intense that even everyday walking becomes difficult. The periods of relief will become shorter, and those of pain longer. Pretty soon, even getting out of bed in the morning and taking the first steps of the day will be excruciatingly painful.

Heelspur syndrome is caused by just that: a bone spur—a mass of bone and calcium deposits actually growing on the heelbone (calcanius)—protruding from the heel. The pain comes from the irritating rub of this extra bone on the tissues surrounding it. If an athlete has all the symptoms of heelspur syndrome, but an x ray reveals no heel spur, acute plantarfascitis, an irritation of that sheetlike muscle which we just described, is usually the culprit.

Whether the pain is caused by a heel spur or acute plantar-fascitis at the heel, the treatment is usually the same: take the pressure off the heel so that the spur won't continue to grow, or the muscle heals itself. The best way to do this is to use some sort of padding in the shoe, either a professional orthotic device, or even a simple horseshoe-shaped foam rubber pad cut to the shape of the heel. The thicker the better: an inch or two of foam rubber will compress as you stand on it, absorbing the shock of walking that your foot usually takes. If foam rubber doesn't work for you, try pads of other shock-absorbing materials: Sorbathane II, Spenco, or PPT. And if one pad isn't enough to ease the pain, use two.

Another simple and useful tactic to use against the pain of heelspurs is to stretch out your calf muscles. Sometimes your rear leg muscles tighten and contract in reaction to a heelspur, because they're trying to lift the heel off the ground faster than normal in reaction to the pain. If you stretch those muscles, you can break the spasm and reduce the pain in your heel.

## ANKLES

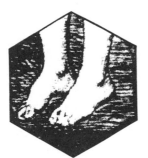

Athlete or not, almost everyone seems to sprain an ankle, that most vulnerable of joints, once in a while. The most frustrating aspect of this common—and very painful—injury is that it is so easily prevented.

You're especially prone to ankle sprains if you turn your ankles inpronate (described in Chapter 1)—as you walk. So the first preventive step we recommend is to determine whether or not you do. Take a look at your oldest pair of shoes. If the insides of the heels are more worn down than the outsides, you're pronating. When you pronate, the ligaments on the outside of the ankle—the ropes of tissue that link the foot bones to each other and hold them in place—tend to shorten up. At the same time, those on the inside are stretched to the limit.

Under these conditions, all it takes is a moment of sudden pressure for the too-taut ligaments to rip.

All it takes for athletes, performing artists, and even sedentary folks—anyone with pronating feet—to prevent ankle sprains is to *stretch*. For athletes and performing artists such as dancers, this stretch should take place as a regular part of your warm-up. Sitting down, cross one ankle over the other knee. Using the hand on the same side of your body as the ankle that's crossed, grasp your ankle just above the ankle bone to hold it steady. Then let your foot relax completely, as loose and limp as it can be.

With the other hand slowly rotate the foot in circles, first in one direction, then the other, for at least thirty seconds each. You'll feel your foot getting warmer and looser. Now gently twist the entire foot inwards at the ankle. This stretches the outside ligaments. Hold it in that position for ten or fifteen seconds, then relax. Again—and be gentle!—twist the foot *out* for ten or fifteen seconds to stretch the outer ligaments. Relax.

Now treat your other ankle to the same "stretch-ercise." The whole procedure takes only three or four minutes, and is well worth it to protect your ankles from sprains and to keep your step springy.

If you're prone to ankle sprains, another good preventive measure—particularly if you're an active sort—is to wear an ankle brace. A simple elastic band, available in drugstores, will give your weak ankle an extra margin of support. Other types of strappings available, and worth investigating, are a modified J-strap for extra support, and air stirrups. The stirrups come with a plastic air bag that helps compress any edema (swelling through water retention) that might recur if you've already sprained your ankle, and are trying to heal it.

Let's say that even though you've taken all these preventive measures, you somehow sprain an ankle. The key to healing is RICE—Rest, Ice, Compression, and Elevation. First, elevate the foot. Then wrap the ankle in an ace bandage and apply ice. Follow the RICE treatment for twenty-four to forty-eight hours. After that, begin—*very* gently—to move and stretch the ankle (continue ice applications to keep down swelling).

That way, your joint will retain its normal range of motion, with minimization of scars and adhesions.

Spraining the same ankle again and again is a sure signal that professional care is necessary. Although most ankle sprains *can* be prevented with stretching before playing or running, a foot imbalance may be present if you sprain the same ankle repeatedly. In that case, a visit to the podiatrist, who may fabricate a professional orthotic device to fit your foot, is in order.

## ACHILLES TENDONS

The Achilles tendon, a strong, ropelike tendon behind the lower half of the lower leg formed by the two tendons that emerge from the two large muscles of the calf (the gastrocnemius and the soleus), extends down the leg, inserting into the heel bone behind the ankle. The Achilles tendon may become inflamed, and can tear at any number of attachment points, usually because one or both of the calf muscles that attach to the tendon is two tight. Although tears and inflammations at specific places along the tendon have more technical names, they are collectively known as Achilles tendonitis.

After a bout with this condition, putting a heel lift in your shoe on the side that was injured can help keep pressure off the tendon. Try at least a quarter-inch of felt or other shock-absorbing material, and be sure it doesn't compress too far. While you're healing, use the lift in *all* your shoes—not just the ones you wear to play. Even walking can irritate the tendon all over again. If you follow these instructions, the tendon should be healed in roughly six weeks.

If you have recurring tendonitis, use the old-shoe test we recommended in the section on ankle sprain to see if you are turning your ankles in—pronating feet can complicate, or even cause, Achilles tendonitis. An orthotic device will help keep your ankles from turning in, and thus keep the tendonitis from *re*turning. At the same time, keep stretching your calf muscles daily. All the muscles in the leg benefit from a warm-up stretch. If they don't get it, they are much more prone to strain while you're playing your sport.

## LOWER LEGS

Like the metatarsals, the lower leg bones are subject to stress fractures. The tibia—the bone that forms the shin—is particularly vulnerable. Because it is thickest in the middle, the upper and lower one-thirds of the bone are especially prone to stress injury. The symptoms of stress fracture here are the same as elsewhere: increased pain as you exercise, decreased pain when you take a break. And treatment is the same, too: rest, ice, and elevation at first, followed by a slow re-entry into play. Build up gradually to your previous intensity and duration when your bones have built up a tolerance for the stress.

A full orthotic—made of a thermoplastic that has been heat-molded to casts of the feet, held as close to their ideal position as possible—can be useful. This controls the foot from heelstrike to toe-off, allowing only normal ranges of motion, rather than the excessive ranges of motion that helped cause the stress fracture. Also, when this device is made with a deep heel cup and a full shock-absorbing insole on top, pressure reduction is achieved, which aids in healing. The orthotic must be worn when walking at *all times*, from the moment you arise from bed to the time you return to bed (with the exceptions of showering, swimming, and walking on a sandy beach). Approximately eight to twelve weeks of full-time use should help effect the healing necessary to resolve a stress fracture.

"Shinsplints" is a layman's term for almost any pain in the front of the lower leg. Although it's a common complaint, there is not really one adequate definition for it. Anterior compartment shinsplints is characterized by inflammation of the muscles and tendons; the swelling in turn presses on nerves and blood vessels, causing pain. *Posterior* compartment shinsplints occurs when muscles pull away from the bone, causing swelling and irritation to the lining of the bone (periostitis).

In either case, a bone scan is the only diagnostic tool that is completely effective. Shinsplints is often misdiagnosed as a stress fracture, and vice versa. One relatively easy way to determine which you have is to pay attention to the pain: a stress fracture generally gets more painful with exercise, while shinsplints often seems to feel better while you're working out, but really awful after you're through.

If you suspect shinsplints, whether in the front or back of your leg, treat the problem with RICE for the first two days, then plenty of stretching and exercise for the rear leg muscles, which are partly to blame in almost every case. Before your re-entry into working out, check with a foot specialist to see whether you have a foot imbalance that could be corrected. Go back to exercising slowly and carefully. And if you've been running on cement, see if you can find a dirt track or grassy area that will accommodate a long run.

Sometimes shinsplints sufferers actually have to resort to surgery for correction. But in ninety-eight percent of cases, such a drastic measure is unnecessary. What *is* necessary to heal shinsplints is plenty of tender loving care, adequate stretching, and a gradual increase in exercise until you're back to your normal routine.

## KNEES AND THIGHS

Now let's touch very broadly on knee and thigh injuries to athletes. Your body operates on the basis of what we call "dynamic equilibrium": for every move you make, there is a muscle or a group of muscles that moves a bone (or bones) in one direction—and another set that pulls in the opposite direction. So *all* your muscles need to be strong.

For example, having highly developed, tight, powerful muscles in the backs of your legs may seem to increase your efficiency as an athlete. But if the muscles in the front of your thighs are weak and stretched out, you may be asking for an injury, because every step you take puts extra stress on your knees and other important joints if your muscles are out of balance. Runner's knee is just one injury that can result from imbalanced strength in the muscles.

In most cases, there is a simple answer to muscle imbalance, and we really can't overemphasize this point: a proper warm-up creates dynamic equilibrium. The leg is then protected, because the muscles are able to hold all the bone structures for proper position for efficient weight-bearing as you move through all the pushes, pulls, ups and downs of a tough athletic workout. And of course, wearing the proper gear for your sport is also a must. If you have a foot or leg imbalance, "proper gear" might include an orthotic device to correct it *before* you get out on the playing field.

# ATHLETICS
# AND
# EXERCISE

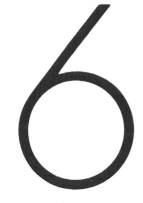

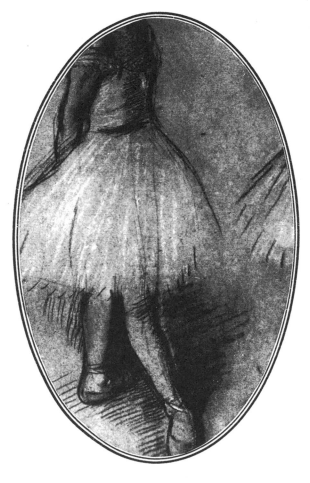

WE'VE COVERED THE basics of foot care from birth to old age. In between, most of us spend a great deal of time on our feet outdoors. We may be athletes, we may simply like to roam on the beach, or we may have discovered the joys of walking as exercise, either on our own or through the advice of our doctors. In this chapter, we are going to address the proper care and maintenance of our feet in exercise programs, whether they be formal athletic programs, plain old fun on the beach, or a walking regime undertaken for exercise.

## ATHLETICS AND AWARENESS: PREVENTING INJURY

All athletics bring the risk of injury, but exercising in itself does not cause injury! Sports injuries almost always result from a lack of awareness—a failure to see the body as a whole.

In Chapter 5 we discussed specific sports-related foot and leg injuries; here we will talk about preventive therapy regimens and a philosophy which balances exercises to maximize their benefits while minimizing their negative stress on the body.

At the same time that the pull of muscles and tendons and the stress of pressure on foot and leg bones drives calcium back into the bones, helping to prevent osteoporosis, that very pressure may lead to stress fractures in the bones of the feet, legs, and, particularly in women, of the pelvis. Thus, balance is crucial in an effective training program. It is important to be in touch with your body not only after but during training to prevent injury. Remember, your body is always giving you feedback. A lack of awareness of this feedback can leave you prone to injury.

You must be aware of your body as a whole, not just as isolated limbs. The upper body has many direct and indirect influences on exercising—a stiff neck or shoulder, for instance, may change the way you twist and move your body, causing an improper angle and pressure on heelstrike which can in turn lead to injuries of the knee, shin and heel bones. A pelvic imbalance can cause one leg to act "shorter" than the other, leading to many of the same injuries. It is a good idea to have your upper body evaluated for biomechanical structural abnormalities and imbalances and to have them treated before you begin training, as well as periodically, to prevent unnecessary injuries.

## CROSS-TRAINING

Cross-training—using two or more sports to balance each other—is one way to ensure training the body as a whole. Cross-training can have a different meaning for each of us, determined by our individual exercise goal. Without these goals clearly defined, there is no clear answer.

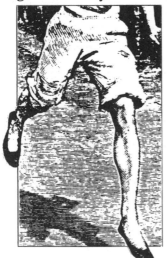

Cross-training for the triathlete often means running, swimming, and cycling. Rowing, skiing, or kayaking are used in some of the more unusual triathlons. However, *any* three aerobic exercises can be part of a triathlon, and one to three sports are practiced daily in preparation for this event.

Cross-training is not only practiced by triathletes; it is a tool used often by athletes to balance their bodies. For a runner, cycling balances the leg by strengthening the anterior leg muscles, which often weaken from jogging. A cyclist may jog to strengthen his rear leg muscles, which weaken from cycling. Balancing the muscles this way increases the stability of joints in the leg and helps prevent injuries to muscles and tendons. Anyone, at any age, can benefit by combining two or more sports. Injuries can be minimized, additional aerobic conditioning gained, stress reduced, and muscle groups rested through alternating exercises. Cross-training also avoids the monotony of training for the same sport over long periods.

It's important to combine exercises that balance each other, however; combinations that work the same muscle groups in similar ways may actually *increase* injury risk. And be sure to start in a careful graduated program. For example, the novice may elect to walk or jog for fifteen minutes and cycle for fifteen minutes at first, increasing each time by about ten percent every two weeks. Never train more than three days in a row; by taking one day of rest the body has a chance to reduce stress buildup and restore energy to the muscles. In fact, beginners may find it easier and safer to alternate days of exercise with days of rest until their strength and endurance grow.

For the trained athlete, practicing only one exercise per day often allows daily exercise, with the elimination of days of rest. But until your body is gradually strengthened by regular training, days of rest are intelligent ideas. And never train past the point of noticeable discomfort—remember, pain is usually a sign of injury.

OVERTRAINING occurs when an athlete has passed his or her peak and is continuing to train at a level that starts to wear away at the body. Careful attention to post-workout weight, the amount of fluid that you take in each day, sleep patterns, and morning heart rate will enable you to be aware of and prevent overtraining. If you start to frequently feel lethargic and tired, you may be overtraining. Constant soreness is another sign that you might have overused parts of your body. Athletes will often tell you that they've had their best performances after an illness, when they've rested and been allowed to heal and reduce stress in their bodies. Be aware: weigh yourself regularly, watching out for rapid weight-loss; make sure you sleep your normal amount; and monitor your resting heart rate to see it stays your normal average.

## WARM-UP AND STRETCHING

The best way to treat muscle and tendon injuries is through prevention, with proper warm-up and stretching. Before we begin stretching muscles or tendons, we have to get them warmed up. The best way to warm up the leg muscles is through the Robins Six Step Exercise:

> Lie down on the ground with your legs straight out in front of you. The exercise must be done with a slow, rhythmic, continuous movement. Counting with a beat, "and-a-one, and-a-two, and-a-three, and-a-four, and-a-five, and-a-six," will give you a proper rhythm for the exercise. It is repeated five or six times in a row on each leg—never alternate legs.
> Step 1: Slowly bring your heel toward you
> Step 2: Bring your knee to your chest, without using your hands
> Step 3: Straighten your leg up in the air so the knee is straight (even if it means lowering the leg slightly)
> Step 4: Lower the straight leg about halfway to the ground
> Step 5: Slowly let your heel come down to the ground
> Step 6: Straighten your leg out again on the ground

This exercise is designed to get the heart rate up slowly and to increase circulation into the muscles.

To prevent most rear leg muscle injuries, use two passive or gentle stretches. First, while you're lying on the ground on your back, using one leg at a time, bring one knee under your leg and help pull your leg and knee into your chest. Never put your hands in front of the knee as they may tend to slide up and can cause the kneecap to jam into the thigh bone and irritate it. When you pull the knee into your chest, it's a long, slow, continuous pull inward, never letting it bounce outward. After twenty seconds (by the clock—all stretches take between ten and thirty seconds) you allow the leg to go straight out again and then repeat the exercise. You should do this three to five times per leg depending on your stiffness. This stretches the hamstring and gluteal muscles, the upper leg muscles. The next stretching exercise is for the calf muscles. This is done by sitting up and grabbing a towel or a belt and slinging it around the bottom of your foot. Grab one end with each hand. Sit with your back and head straight and your arms straight out in front of you, holding the belt or towel. Do not let your arms bend at the elbow joint. Now, lean backwards and allow your body weight to pull your foot toward you. After that, let go of the towel with one hand and your foot should flop forward to the level where the other foot is resting, if you weren't using muscle power to pull the foot towards you. This exercise should be repeated three to five times per leg depending upon injury and tightness.

The two best post-exercise stretches are two active stretches. The first one is the "against-the-wall stretch." This is for the lower rear leg muscles. Stand as close to the wall as you can get, facing it, feet and legs a shoulder-width apart, palms held on the wall, face-level or higher. Take a step back, keeping both your feet pointing perpendicular to the wall. In the first against-the-wall stretch, the rear leg is kept straight. Don't force your hips forward when you lean into the stretch and hyperextend your knee. Try to keep your rear leg, knee, hip and shoulder all in a straight line. Now, lean into the wall and support yourself with your entire arm and forearm. Hold this position for twenty seconds. You should feel the stretch from behind the knee all the way down into the heel. Hold it for twenty seconds, push out away from the wall to relax the stretch. Do not allow your heel to come off the ground during stretching. In the second against-the-wall stretch, allow the rear leg to bend slightly forward at the knee. This works another portion of the lower rear leg muscles. You will feel the stretch more in the belly of the calf muscle and down behind the heel bone. This should be performed three to five times per leg with no alternation of legs.

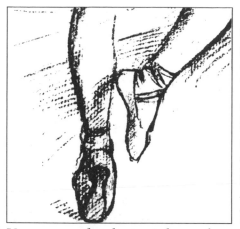

The next most important muscles to stretch actively are the hamstring muscles, the upper rear leg muscles. This stretch, the "sleepwalker stretch" is performed by placing your foot on a chair, a stool or a table, straightening your leg that's placed on this table and pulling your foot very forcefully towards your body and holding it that way. Keep your back straight and arms straight out in front of you. Let your fingertips rise gently as you lean forward gently. By lifting your fingertips up and your arms up as you lean forward you will find that your back stays straight, thus putting no pressure on it; pulling your foot forcefully towards you with muscle power will create a strong stretch on the rear leg muscles.

There is a special stretch for ileotibial band syndrome. In this stretch you stand with your shoulder leaning against the wall and step away from the wall with both feet. Then gently let your hip lean in towards the wall. This causes your body to move in the shape of the letter C gently stretching the ileotibial band in the leg. This is performed three to five times per leg. It is not necessary to perform this stretch often if you have no symptoms of ileotibial band syndrome.

While most athletes tend to stretch too little, which causes tight muscles and tendons, leading to potential injury, overstretching also can result in injury. A stretch is defined as a slow, continuous pull on muscle and tendon. It should last for a minimum of ten to as much as thirty seconds. There should never be any bouncing motion as this can tighten the muscle and tendon. When a person stretches for over thirty seconds per repetition the muscle and tendon fiber elongate past their ideal length, causing a laxity which can lead to injury. Stretching a cold, unwarmed-up muscle and tendon can also overstretch it.

## THERAPIES TO PREVENT AND HEAL INJURY

Daily massage is a wonderful way to help eliminate injuries and prevent tightness in muscles after exercising. Any form of massage is beneficial; two massage routines for the feet and legs are described in Chapter 8. More advanced techniques, like shiatsu and acupressure can be used regularly to speed recovery time and eliminate minor stresses in muscles and tendons, but require more training.

Orthotics, devices worn in shoes to rebalance foot structure, thus helping to maintain the integrity of the entire leg and body structure, are necessary for a small group of people; this subject is discussed more fully in Chapter 7. Professional evaluation by a sports podiatrist will reveal hidden problems that may require these devices, before injuries result. Specifically developed sports devices are also necessary for some sports used in cross training. Ankle braces—whether tape, elastic bands, pneumatic braces, or gel training braces—can prevent reinjury to weak ankles.

Electromagnetic therapy, the newer version of magnetic therapy (which uses round magnets), can have spectacular results. For injuries in muscles and bones the north side of magnets have been used for years to help heal the injured part. In more recent times machines which convert low-voltage electricity into magnetic energy have been employed. Animal and human studies have shown that by pulsing (electronically turning the magnetic field on and off rapidly) the magnetic field generates a powerful safe healing action. This takes place by reducing the buildup of protein molecules that cluster between cells in an injured or painful area. Breaking up these clusters of protein molecules allows for a normal flow of lymph (water) in and out of the injured or painful area. This reduces swelling and pain, allowing for a return of normal blood and lymph circulation to the area, which promotes healing.

In our clinical experience, we found that this has its most astonishing effect on any bone injury or problem. It has dramatically shortened the healing time of fractures, stress fractures, bone bruises, and joint injuries and inflamations. It has also been effective in treating muscle injuries, arthitis, and many other problems. Only trained professionals should employ pulsed electromagnetic therapy, however; the healing effect can be reversed by using the wrong settings. Stationary magnets are much safer for home use, as you simply place the north pole against the injured or painful body part.

Whirlpool baths and hot baths help increase blood circulation to muscles, relaxing them. And last, but not least, mental visualization techniques for relaxation and healing can speed recovery time and help prevent injuries, as well as to improve athletic performance. The mind is the most powerful part of our body, but we usually call on only a fraction of its potential ability. For many years people have been taught to mentally visualize various movements to help them perform assigned tasks. This concentration concept was carried over into athletic training. Studies have shown that when people imagine themselves performing a work task or athletic movement perfectly, their performance of the task or movement improves greatly in speed, accuracy, and repetition, with fewer injuries occuring.

We have employed the same concept in healing. The first step is to visualize the painful or injured body part. Some knowledge of internal anatomy is necessary, or you must glance through an anatomy textbook. By mentally "sighting" what the internal injury looks like, layer by layer (even down to cellular levels), you can then call on your mind to effect the healing changes that are necessary.

This exercise should be performed three to four times a day for five minutes. It is important not to try and mentally "force" the healing. Try and stay at ease, completely relaxed during the healing session. Repeat the process daily until healed.

## RECREATION FOR THE NON-ATHLETE

For those of you who are not athletes, we have plenty of good advice for when you do find yourself playing outdoors, especially in the summer.

THE BEACH    Maybe one of your favorite summer sports is to run along the beach. Good exercise, perhaps, and it's certainly exhilarating to run in sand under a hot sun, but the situation can be *disastrous*, not only for your feet, but also for your legs, lower back, hips, and knees. Sand, especially deep, thick sand, will allow the foot to move in any direction. By running in sand you are inviting your feet to pronate, supinate, twist in, or twist out, throwing off your whole leg and possibly your lower back as well. In other words, you're asking for an injury.

Let's say you're running on the wetter sand, near the water. Your foot's not going to twist, because you're on firmer ground. But if you're running near the water, you're running on an incline. One leg actually acts as if it's shorter than the other, because the limb and pelvis are raised on one side. Even if you run back in the other direction, you're still running with one short leg. Again, you are inviting injury and pain to your lower back, knee, hip, and pelvis. So unless you find the ideal beach—one with flat, wet sand—running on the beach is not the best exercise.

On the other hand, swimming is great exercise for the legs and feet. Even if you can't swim, just walking waist-deep into the water and jumping up and down when the waves roll in is an excellent way to help strengthen and tone up the muscles in your legs, as well as work you out aerobically. Ideally, you should swim or jump for twenty minutes at a stretch.

Although most of us are very careful about applying sunscreens to our upper body and legs at the beach, our poor feet often go forgotten. It's important to protect both the tops *and* bottoms of your feet, particularly if you are lying on your stomach in the sun. And if you're walking up and down the shoreline, remember that the water reflects a great deal of light onto your lower legs. Again, be protected. And of course, always reapply your sunscreen after a swim.

It's fun to walk barefoot on the beach, yet that fun can be cut short by a splinter, piece of glass, or sharp shell in your foot. It's a good idea to wear some kind of sandal while walking or beachcombing to protect your feet against a sudden and painful surprise. Sandals or thongs will also protect you from hot sand, which can quickly burn the soles of your feet. If you just can't give up walking barefoot in the sand, at least keep your eyes on the ground, for the sake of your feet! Then you can avoid potentially dangerous situations, such as sharp or rusty foreign objects and deep holes. And if you're going to walk on the sand—with or without sandals—walk slowly and relax. Don't overexert yourself in the heat, and drink plenty of liquids to keep yourself from becoming dehydrated.

When you're home from the beach, it's time to treat your feet and legs to moisture. The sun dries out your skin drastically, literally cooking the skin's elastin. If you don't add some oil—in the form of a moisturizer—to the skin on your feet and legs now, you'll lose some of the suppleness there that protects you against cuts, bruises, and other injuries.

**COUNTRY WALKS**    Another favorite summertime sport is walking in the country. Sounds benign enough. But for the city dweller, a country terrain poses all kinds of unexpected danger to the feet and legs. First, watch the terrain under your feet. Sticks and stones *may* break your bones if your head is in the stars and the sticks and stones are under your feet. Watch where you are going!

Second, dress properly. Try to avoid wearing shorts in the woods, which are full of poison ivy, poison sumac, poison oak, and other irritants. It's a smart idea to know what these plants look like, as well, so that you can avoid them. Wear good thick cotton socks, and either a pair of athletic shoes, or hiking boots. If you're going to be out for a while, powder your feet carefully, and take an extra pair of socks along to keep the powder (and your feet) dry. Warm sweat is the perfect medium in which to develop athlete's foot.

If your walk includes a sojourn by a bubbling brook or a lake, remember to apply sunscreen to your feet when you take your shoes off, as you would on the beach. And if a swim is on the agenda, follow the same rules we outlined above about going barefoot and reapplying sunscreen afterwards. You might want to take an extra precaution if you're going into the lake: wear your thongs to prevent cutting your feet on what may be resting on the lake's bottom.

**GOLF**  So you're a summer golfer? If you're walking the course for the first time of the season, go easy on yourself. Get used to it slowly, even if that means *not* shooting eighteen holes the first day. A relaxed attitude means less tension for your feet and legs, which in and of itself helps prevent injury or strain. Warm up with some stretching exercises. On the other hand, if you plan to use a golf cart, try to get some walking in, or the exercise value of your afternoon will be zero.

**TENNIS AND OTHER ACTIVE SPORTS**  If your summer game is tennis or another racket sport, or volleyball, the important thing is to warm up first. With these more active sports, it is also important to consider our advice to athletes above about how to avoid injury and treat it when it occurs. If you're going to be playing under a hot summer sun, drink plenty of liquid to avoid dehydration. Water is best—and the colder the better. Second, if you're going to be playing for a while, have a spare pair of socks—and even shoes—to cut the chances of fungus infections and athlete's foot growing in a damp, warm, sweaty environment.

**HORSEBACK RIDING**  Especially if you ride only once in a blue moon, proper footgear is absolutely essential—with *heels*, so that you can keep your feet in the stirrups. You should also have some kind of shock absorption in your shoes or boots, since riding a horse can be jarring on the feet. Insoles made of a protective material such as foam rubber, PPT, or Sorbathane are appropriate here. Such protection will help cushion the bouncing and jarring of the ride, preventing ankle and knee discomfort, as well as injury to the hips.

## WALKING AS EXERCISE

Walking has only recently been recognized as an excellent exercise for everyone, properly done. For those of us who just can't seem to throw ourselves into the more active forms of exercise—running, swimming, or cycling—a good walking exercise program can be, quite literally, a life-saver. But let's make it clear that we are talking about a walking *exercise* program here—and not just the garden-variety walking that most of us do every day. To condition our heart and circulation, tone up our muscles, and generally keep our body systems functioning at optimum capacity, walking has to be undertaken systematically and conscientiously. It must be done daily: as a conditioning program it is not as efficient as the cross-training program described above, which could be done two or three times a week. If you're elderly or out of shape, however, you might start your program by walking for three or four days in a row, and then taking a day off to let your body rest.

**BUILDING UP A WALKING PROGRAM**   As with any other exercise program, embark on a walking routine in a gradual, systematic way. You have to build up the length of time that you walk, from perhaps ten minutes a day at the beginning of your program, to thirty minutes or an hour when you're in shape.

A big help in starting your walking exercise program is to keep a notebook of your progress. As in other forms of aerobic exercise, progress is measured by pulse rate. First, establish what your optimum heart rate for exercise should be: start with the number 220, subtract your age from it, and

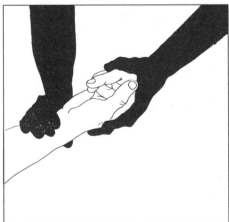

multiply that result by sixty to seventy-five percent. This target pulse rate will serve as a goal for your walking program. Next, test your pulse rate while you are sitting down. The best place to take your pulse is at your wrist or temple. If you use your wrist, use all the lesser fingertips to feel the pulse. Never use your thumb; it has an artery with a pulse strength that can interfere with your reading. The fingertips are placed on either of the two grooves found on the underside of the wrist near the outer edges (see diagram). You may take your pulse for a minute, or as little as ten seconds (remember to multiply by six to get the number of beats per minute). Never take your pulse at your neck (the carotid pulse) because unless you use very gentle pressure you can slow your pulse rate down by triggering the carotid sinus reflex, which acts directly on the heart. Record your pulse number in your notebook.

As you walk, stop every five or ten minutes and take your pulse again. This will give you some idea of the effect the exercise is having on your heartbeat and circulation, and how close you are getting to your target pulse rate. When you get home from your walk, record the highest pulse rate reached during exercise in your notebook.

An important aspect of the walking exercise program is that you not only increase the *length* of your daily walk on a systematic basis, you also increase the *speed* of your walk. Why? With increased exercise, your heart rate will tend to decrease. Therefore, to reach the desired goal, you must exert yourself to increase the challenge to your heart and circulation. If you are elderly or disabled you may be unable to do this; in that case, compensate by increasing the length of time you walk, even to one or two hours a day. The longer (and faster) you walk, the more conditioning you're going to get.

Build up slowly, in terms of both time and pace, to a peak program. If you're using time as your guide, add about ten percent more to the time you walk every two weeks: that is, if you start by walking twenty to thirty minutes a day, after two weeks add two or three minutes, and so on. If distance is your guide, increase it too by roughly ten percent every two weeks. This allows for safe stress buildup in the bones and muscles, and lets the heart adapt to the stress that's suddenly being placed on it. Remember to use your notebook!

**GETTING READY**   What you wear is important. You should wear a comfortable, well-fitting shoe that will cushion and protect your feet—a running shoe is ideal, since it's made for the same unidirectional motion as walking. What you *don't* wear is as important as what you do. Don't carry anything— not even a purse, if you can help it. Any weight at all can throw your posture off and impede your walk. Try to wear clothing that will allow for heat buildup to dissipate as quickly and as comfortably as possible. Cotton undergarments are important because they allow the moisture on your body to evaporate.

Running shirts and jogging pants are good to walk in, as long as they are made of materials that will absorb and dissipate perspiration. In the winter your outer clothing should be made of wool, which "breathes" while keeping you warm, while the clothing next to your skin should be cotton or polypropylene—and wear something to keep your face warm, as well as gloves or mittens.

It's best to walk on a somewhat empty stomach. Try not to eat for two or three hours before walking, just so your body won't be burdened by trying to digest a meal and walking at the same time. However, you should be completely hydrated before you start—drink eight to ten ounces of water every hour before you go. This precautionary measure ensures that your body won't overheat as fast while you're walking.

A warm-up is essential, just as in any other exercise program. The first step here is to relax—body and mind—for at least five to ten minutes. Try to let any tension or anxiety go. This prepares the ground for loosening up your muscles.

Now that you've relaxed, warm up for five or ten minutes. This warm-up could be a simple exercise like just walking in place indoors until you feel that your blood has started circulating at a faster rate—or try Dr. Robins's Six Step Exercise, described earlier in this chapter. Then loosen up: move all your joints, from the neck down: the shoulders, the elbows, the wrists, the fingers, the hips, and the knees.

When you get to your feet, spend at least a minute on each one, massaging it, kneading it, and flexing all the joints by hand. This prepares your feet to take the burden and the brunt of a good walk. Because it helps them to respond to stress more readily, it's a great preventive measure against injuries.

*Plan your route* before you go: determine just where you're going to be walking, what kind of terrain you are going to encounter. Avoid areas of rough terrain, or streets that have been broken up. You'll want to concentrate on your walking—not on avoiding potholes!

**GOOD WALKING STYLE**   So your walk has finally begun. The first thing to be aware of is your posture, an integral part of this exercise program. You should be erect, with your head up, shoulders back, chest out, stomach in. Try to avoid being slumped, stoop-shouldered, or hunchbacked. Don't look straight down at the ground; you can see the ground out a few steps in front of you by looking straight ahead. Remember, whichever direction the head goes, the rest of the body follows. By keeping your back straight, your spine elongated, and your head up in the air, you're giving your spine a good stretch, which reduces pressure on the vertebra, the legs, and the feet.

Walk with a regular cadence, at a speed that's most comfortable, to begin with. Walking at a slower rate to start helps warm your body up. After five or ten minutes of walking slowly, you can work up gradually to the actual speed you want to maintain. There's no need to take big, long steps, which can actually throw you off balance and cause an accident. Instead, increase the cadence—the number of steps you take—to raise your heart rate.

At the beginning of your walk, as you are building up to the rate of speed you'd like to maintain for awhile, you may have lots of energy. When you feel winded or tired, feel free to slow down to a comfortable pace. This builds up your wind, restoring your tissues by getting more fresh blood into them to wash away waste products and build up the energy flow. When you feel stronger and less winded, you can step up your pace once more. By varying the pace of your walk depending on how you feel, you'll find that you actually get into shape faster. At that point you can maintain the faster speed for longer periods of time. Again, keeping your notebook is important so that you can see your progress clearly.

As you walk, a natural swing of the arms from front to back is important. Not too tight, not too loose, is the rule: for example, never hold your hand in a tight fist, but don't let it fall totally slack at your side, either. Just hold your fingers lightly together, with the thumb resting on top of the index finger. If your arms are swinging the way we described, your shoulders will be relaxed as well.

As far as the lower half of your body goes, you should be swinging your legs from the hips forward, allowing the heel to strike the ground before the ball of the foot, slightly on the outside. If you find yourself bouncing up and down, walking on your toes, your rear leg muscles probably need to be stretched. But it is better to do that *after* you walk, rather than before or during your exercise.

The way you breathe is important to the way you walk. Abdominal breathing is best: breathe through your nose, and let the breath go out through your mouth. Take long, deep breaths that fill up the upper and lower portion of your lungs. This type of breathing naturally forces your stomach to expand when you inhale: hence the name, "abdominal breathing." When you exhale, you can actually also see your stomach expand a little. Breathing this way gets the most oxygen possible into your system quickly, increasing your strength and stamina during the exercise.

If you start to get winded and feel that you have to breathe a little faster, by all means, breathe faster. If you get so winded that you have to stop, don't fight it. Stop. Take a few deep, cleansing breaths to reoxygenate your body tissues. Then continue with your walk. This is especially important if you have a lung problem or heart trouble. (We'll talk more about specific guidelines for people with heart trouble in the next few pages.)

What if you develop cramps in your legs while you're walking? Stop. Massage the muscle and let the cramp dissipate. Then continue walking. If you then feel the cramp starting to build again, stop again. Cramps may be caused by the waste products building up in the muscles without enough oxygen and blood to wash them away. By massaging the ailing tissues, you help break up some of the spasm in the muscle fibers and increase the circulation. By doing that, you help wash away the waste products, which reenergizes these tissues cells, allowing you to continue your walk free of pain.

**AFTER THE WALK** After your daily walk, the most important muscles to stretch are the muscles in front of your leg, since they may actually be weak- ened by walking. Now's the time to do the belt exercise and the "against-the- wall" exercise (described earlier in this chapter) to relax your *rear* leg muscles 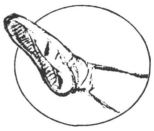 before strengthening the ones in the front. Then, for your front leg muscles, sit on a countertop, or firm table top. Slowly extend your foot up in front of you, until your leg is perfectly straight out. You should be in an L shape, with your back straight. Hold that for ten seconds and let your leg come back down to a bent knee position. Repeat this from ten to twenty times for each leg, as you develop your strength. (You can use a light ankle weight—either storebought or home- made—but it shouldn't really be necessary if you're walking every day.)

After you walk, it is also important to rehydrate your system by drinking plenty of fluid. If you don't do this, you may feel very weak, and blame your weakness on the exer- cise, when it really stems from dehydration. You may also want to eat a light meal after your pulse rate returns to its normal sedentary pace.

**THE BENEFITS OF A WALKING PROGRAM** By walking in this way, consciously and with discipline, not only are you benefiting the entire muscular system of the body, you are also burning excess fat and reducing overall body weight; gaining balance, stamina, strength, and endurance; improving cardiovascular fitness by improving your overall circulation; and, in the process, increasing your ability to relax emotion- ally—the extra oxygen to the brain raises the levels of sere- tonin and endorphin, morphine-like substances that allow a state of relaxation—even euphoria—to occur.

After a year of walking aerobically—increasing your pulse rate during exercise and increasing the supply of oxygen to your body—you should see noticeable changes in your cardio-vascular system, in your alertness and muscle tone, and also in your reflex action. You will have more stamina, strength, and endurance. This walking program is one of the best ways available of slowing down the aging process to its normal level, and improving overall foot and leg health at the same time. It is an important step on the road to health.

An interesting note for dieters: recent studies have determined that if you are exercising at seventy to seventy-five percent of your maximum heart rate, you are taking in enough oxygen to burn fat more rapidly than any other fuel source available. (See the section entitled "Building Up a Walking Program" to calculate this figure.) Your body will turn to the fat as fuel very rapidly, using it for about seventy percent of the energy it needs to exercise. If you work up to over seventy to seventy-five percent of your maximum heart rate, your body will turn to the glycogen (starch) stored in the muscles and tissues, and start to burn that up as well. The oxygen ratios are very difficult to determine for different individuals, and we won't go into it in any further detail here; but if you want to lose weight through this (or any other) exercise program, try to get yourself up to that seventy or seventy-five percent target rate.

**SPECIAL ADVICE FOR HEART PATIENTS** If you have a heart condition, have yourself thoroughly checked out by your doctor or cardiologist to determine whether or not a walking exercise program is safe for you. Although walking as exercise is frequently recommended by doctors for heart patients, some individuals (arthritics, for example) may be advised not to embark on a gravity form of exercise. These people may be able to undertake a walking exercise program in a swimming pool, however, where the pull of gravity is less of a consideration. The water reduces their body weight, yet the resistance of the water also makes an aerobic challenge for the heart and circulation.

If you are participating in a "walking" exercise program in a pool, remember to warm up. You can warm up in the pool itself—hold on to the side of the pool, allowing your feet to rise in light stretches and other movements that will loosen up your muscles. Then walk in place in a shallow part of the pool.

If you have had a heart attack and your doctor approves a walking exercise program on the ground, be sure to keep your face covered with a scarf or mask in cold weather. It is also a wise idea to carry with you a vial of nitroglycerin in case of angina. Be sure that your medicine is in a place where you can reach it *fast*.

**OTHER SPECIAL SITUATIONS**    If you are used to a walking exercise program at sea level or lower, and you vacation in the mountains, be prepared for a change in your pace and time. Because there is less oxygen at higher altitudes, you may find that your heart rate changes because, quite simply, you are working harder. Your heart has to work harder to pump more blood through the body, since there is less oxygen in the blood to transport. Also, the heart has to transport the blood more quickly to be as effective in delivering the same amount of oxygen to the muscles as it does at lower levels of altitude. So don't be surprised if your normal pace and time don't hold up in the mountains. Work up gradually to what you consider a reasonable speed and distance.

As we have already discussed, for various reasons, walking on the beach is not a good idea. Nor is walking around a track, just because walking in circles hurts your knees. However, you should establish your own particular "track," free from obstacles, as this makes your walking program predictable and easier to follow on a daily basis.

If winter weather is too much of an obstacle for you, or you have a heart problem that prohibits exercise in the cold, try walking indoors. Especially if you have a long hall in which you can walk "laps," this can be almost as effective as an outdoor walking exercise program. Remember to keep your notebook, and increase your speed and distance regularly. If you don't have a long hall, you can follow a snakelike "track" within your house, determining what a "lap" is, and increasing your speed and distance accordingly.

Walking up and down stairs can be beneficial if you want to increase your conditioning potential. Be warned, however, that this exercise can lead to muscle imbalances, tightening up of the rear leg muscles and weakening the muscles in front. Thus, you will have to compensate with exercise and stretching therapy to stretch the rear leg muscles and strengthen the front ones. Also, the added shock of the height of the stairs can lead to knee, hip, and low back problems. If you are vulnerable to injury in any of those places, avoid taking your walking exercise on the stairs. If you *are* going to walk up and down stairs, do it only after a proper warm-up.

The same (and more) goes for walking up hills. Be properly warmed up, and also be aware that hills call for a different style of walking. You should lean forward as you walk up and down the hill, relaxing and taking shorter steps than you would take when walking on level ground. Let your arms swing more than usual to help you get up the hill better, and to help you relax as you stride down the hill. This takes some of the pressure off your legs, which have to work harder to resist the pull of gravity.

# FOOTWEAR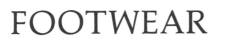

**7**

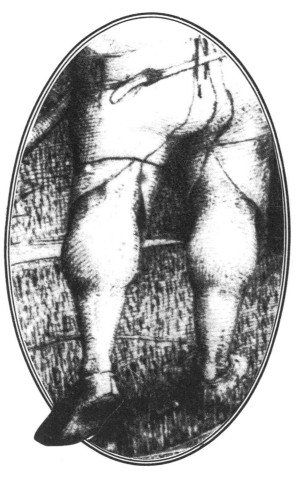

# BUYING A SHOE

SHOES ARE A complicated subject. The first rule is simple: "If the shoe fits, wear it." But what the word "fits" means is *not* so simple, as we shall see.

**FIT**   First, decide what kind of shoe you really need—where you are going to wear it, what you are going to do in it. It doesn't pay to buy a high-style dress shoe for long-distance walking, nor is it appropriate to buy a walking shoe for dress wear. Shoes that you're going to be spending very little time walking in can be purchased with appearance and style, more than comfort, in mind. There's certainly nothing wrong with a fashionable shoe, as long as you don't plan to do much walking in it. Fit the shoe to the occasion; next, find a shoe that will fit your feet.

The first rule here is the "rule of thumb": you should have at least a thumbnail's length between the end of your longest toe and the end of the shoe. This ensures adequate toe room, which lessens your chances of developing toenail or toe irritations because your shoes are too short. Remember, your foot slides forward from an eighth to a quarter of an inch each time you take a step in a shoe, so that thumbnail's-length is important. If you don't have it, you're going to jam your toes into the end of your shoes.

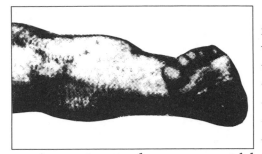

The next thing to look for is adequate width. The width of your foot is usually measured across the ball of the foot, from the bunion joint to the little toe. The easiest way to tell whether or not the shoe you're trying is the proper width for your foot is to do this: stand up, take your thumb and roll it across the leather, across the ball of the foot from one side to the other. You should be able to see the leather wave, almost as if you could pinch it between your thumb and forefinger if you wanted to, but not quite. That's a good test to use to determine if you have an adequate amount of width. If your bunion joints or little toe joints press out on the shoe when you're standing up, and the shoe doesn't have this kind of give to it, it's too tight. Too-tight shoes can lead to bunion or little-toe irritations and corns and calluses. So make sure you have enough room in the width.

The next thing to look for is that the shoe fits the width of your heel. Most good shoes are made with what are called "combination lasts," wider up front and narrower in the heels, which is just what most feet need. Cheaper shoes are made without this combination lasting, so they wind up slipping off the heel or fitting improperly in the front to make the heel stick. It's better to avoid cheap shoes: you'll usually end up jimmying them up in some way to make them fit your foot, and it's just not worth the money or the discomfort to buy a shoe that doesn't fit properly to start.

Now look to see that there is adequate height in the front of the shoe. The top of the shoe shouldn't rub against toes that are higher than the others because they're hammered or slightly raised. If the shoe rubs, you're inviting corns on the tops of your toes. Also make sure that, if the shoe is leather (which is preferable), the leather is soft enough to bend and flex with the foot easily. A leather shoe that doesn't give will irritate your foot.

**MATERIALS AND CONSTRUCTION**    A leather upper will let your foot breathe inside the shoe, allowing perspiration to escape, as well as drying out properly overnight. Cotton has the same advantages, although it doesn't give your foot as much support. As far as the insole and inner materials go, the more natural the better. Synthetic materials can cause your feet to heat up within the shoe, leading to a buildup of perspiration which can cause problems for your feet as well as accelerate the breakdown of your shoes.

While leather soles used to be considered ideal (for the same reasons that leather uppers are preferable), thick rubber soles, or soles made of a synthetic material, are more shock-absorbing for the hard surfaces that we have to walk on. They save wear-and-tear on your feet in a way that leather simply can't. Of course if you're going to be mostly sitting in your shoes, then a thin leather sole can be quite elegant. The soles and heels of shoes can be repaired almost indefinitely, so as long as you pay attention to *when* they need to be repaired, those parts of the shoe are made to last you very well indeed. The upper part of your shoes, however, is less easily repaired. So *before* you purchase your shoes, check to see that the upper is well-made.

The back part of the upper, the part that surrounds the heel and comes along the side of the foot about midway forward, is called the *counter*. The counter is usually made of a rigid material—nowadays, some form of plastic. Look for a rigid, firm counter. The cheaper counters, which are made out of stitched leather or cheaper plastic, tend to give and break very easily. Remember, in dress shoes, as well as regular walking shoes, you really need a good, firm counter, not just because the shoe will last you longer, but also because your foot needs the support that only a well-made counter will give. Most good running shoes have very firm counters, as do most orthopedic shoes.

Another component of a pair of shoes is a steel shank that runs along the bottom, extending from just underneath the heel to the ball of the foot. There is no way you can *see* this shank when you're buying a pair of shoes, so it's best to buy good quality shoes, because you can then assume that the shank is strong and will not bend out of shape easily. In addition, the shoe will give your foot better support if the quality of the shank is good.

Heels should never be totally flat. Even Alexander the Great put heels on the sandals of his troops, because he found that they could march longer distances with heels than without them. A heel height of approximately one inch, with a slight wedge construction, gives the average person the best prevention against leg, foot, and lower-back problems, especially if the shoe is to be used for walking.

Women tend to go too high in their heel height. High-heeled dress shoes can be beautiful, but need to be balanced out with the proper stretching exercises after you wear them, or they tend to shorten the calf muscles, hamstrings, and buttocks, which can lead to lower-back, knee, and ankle trouble. If you aren't going to take the time to stretch your feet and legs properly after wearing high heels, it's best to just stick to one- to one-and-a-half inch heels. You'll be saving yourself a lot of pain, and possibly medical bills as well. High heels for men have never been all that fashionable in our culture, but the short men who use high heels to make themselves taller will encounter the same difficulties that women who wear high heels do, unless, of course, they counteract the side effects of high heels with proper stretching.

Whether the heels of your shoes are made of leather or rubber makes only a little difference. A rubber heel has the slight advantage of absorbing more stress when the heel strikes the ground, when the body may be taking as much as 2.4 times its own weight in force. So a rubber heel on a walking shoe is something of a boon.

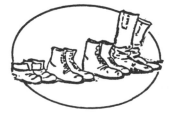

**STYLE** Slip-on shoes are better for dress wear, whereas strap and lace shoes, which don't allow the foot to move around in the shoe quite so much, are probably better walking shoes. If you walk a lot on the job, you're better off in an oxford of some sort rather than a slip-on.

Boots, as far as we're concerned, are basically meant for dress wear. They should be used for limited walking, because they just don't hold the foot to the shoe securely. The movement they allow can lead to instability and therefore problems, especially if you have a structural imbalance in your foot or leg to begin with. When buying a boot, it's best to give yourself a shade less than the thumbnail's-length you normally need between the end of your toe and the end of the boot, so as to give your foot a little less room to move around in the boot when you walk. Too much room in a boot is bound to create rubbing and blisters. On the other hand, as with any other kind of shoe, if you don't give your foot *enough* room, you're going to develop corns on your toes, or your bunion joints are going to be irritated. Our recommendations concerning heel height apply here as well; one-and-a-half inches is ideal. If you're going to be wearing those very dressy boots with three- or four-inch heels, be sure to stretch after you wear them.

As we said, boots are for dress wear. Contrary to the popular song, they aren't "made for walking." But if you insist on wearing boots full-time, you might just be able to pull it off if you're a cowboy out West, or a farmer—someone who walks mostly on soft earth. In those cases boots probably make sense, and they might even be comfortable, without the stress of walking on concrete in the city.

Sandals are meant for the beach. Sandals are meant for pools. Sandals are not really meant to be used on hard surfaces. The same goes for moccasins and deck shoes—they are just not meant for walking on streets. They were made for softer earth, for casual living in the suburbs or in the country. They're great for camping trips. But in the city, they don't do your feet or your body any justice at all. They transmit huge amounts of stress and force into your feet that can really *hurt* them. Save your sandals for the beach, your deck shoes for the boat, and your moccasins for the country.

The same goes for ballet slippers and exercise sandals. It seems to be fashionable right now to wear these on the street; maybe they feel comfortable. But you're not doing your feet any favors by wearing these shoes out of their milieu. You're letting your feet splay more than they're used to, and while that might feel comfortable, or even be good for your feet for limited periods of time at home or on soft ground, it is *not* good on concrete surfaces.

Rubber thongs should definitely be confined to beach or pool, and even there, they can present problems. The synthetics used in them can cause skin irritation when they react with the perspiration from your feet. At the beach, they can catch in the sand, and you can end up with a twisted ankle. The thongs between your toes can cause blisters, so it's best to use a little moleskin, a band-aid, or some cotton on them. These shoes are basically in the "wear at your own risk" category.

Another "wear-at-your-own-risk" shoes is the earth shoe. When it first came out, the earth shoe and its imitators were touted as *the* answer to foot and leg trouble. It had what was called a negative heel, a heel lower than the front of the shoe, in a reverse wedge. This put wearers—particularly women who had been wearing high heels—at a great disadvantage. The result was that a lot of people developed Achilles tendonitis—inflammation of the Achilles tendon behind the heel, as well as pain in the calves, hamstrings, hips and lower back. More seriously, complete tearing of the achilles tendon warranted surgery for some people. All the wearer had to do was step off the curb or walk down a flight of stairs or step out of a car or bus. The heel would come down even further on strike, stretching the calf muscle to the limit.

The earth shoe fad died a natural death; to give it due credit, however, it did help popularize a natural-shaped shoe front. Until then, shoes had been made to stylize the shape of the foot. While the earth shoe wasn't very flattering to the feet, it did fit the shapes of people's feet, rather than expecting the shapes of people's feet to mold into it. As a result, a much wider variety of shoes now actually take the shape of the human foot into account—Clarke's popular "Wallaby" style comes to mind here.

The ideal walking shoe, standing shoe, and everyday shoe is the running shoe. This applies to just about everybody, runners or not. Only a few specialized structural problems do not benefit from the running shoe. For one thing, running shoes are more shock-absorbing than the average leather shoe, or any other kind of sports shoe. They are built with a wedge. They are meant for unidirectional motion, rather than multidirectional motion. The wide-flared heel gives good ankle and knee stability by preventing the foot from moving around inside the shoe. Running shoes shock-absorb the forefoot as well as the heelstrike, thus reducing the amount of pressure that will go through the foot and leg. This reduces lower-back, hip, and knee pain that can develop from stress and pressure on the feet and legs.

More and more people are taking to the running shoe. They wear them for walking to work and then, if need be, change into a dressier shoe which they've carried with them. In New York we see models, executives of corporations, secretaries, and women who work in boutiques dressed to the teeth for their jobs—but on their feet are running shoes. Nothing better has ever happened to city-dwellers' feet.

## SHOES FOR WORK

The best shoe to wear to work is a shoe that best fits your needs on the job. This seems obvious, but it's quite difficult for people to understand that certain shoes are totally inappropriate to protect their feet at work.

First, you must consider what your feet and body do at work—are you mostly sitting, standing, or walking, or all three? Next, what kind of surface are you working on—carpeting or concrete? Finally, take your individual foot's structure—narrow or wide, rigid or flexible—into account.

As an example, a chef in a restaurant stands for many hours, and moves in many directions. His shoe should be shock absorbing, flexible and high in support; but it must have a heel which allows multidirectional movement, so a running shoe is not appropriate. A basketball or tennis sneaker is flexible, shock absorbing and supportive, and would best fit the bill here. A construction worker also needs flexibility and shock absorption, but he also needs protection from injury, in the form of a steel toe. His best bet is to use a shock-absorbing insole inside a steel-toed work shoe—and there needs to be enough room in the shoe for this insole.

Those who stand still on the job need a shock-absorbing shoe that is very stable to give support to the ankle and leg. A running shoe's wide heel provides this stability; certain work shoes, which have rubber or crepe soles and very strong counters at the rear, are also good choices.

## SHOES FOR SPORTS

Shoes for sports have been getting better and better in the last ten or twelve years. Spurred by joggers and runners all over the world, shoe manufacturers are competing to improve the shock-absorbing qualities, flexibility, lightness, and support mechanisms of running shoes. In the process so much has been learned about how the feet move, and what they need to do it properly, that shoes for other sports have benefited as well. Sports shoes are getting lighter and lighter, while maintaining their ability to absorb shock and to flex with the feet. In addition, they are becoming better suited to the particular sport for which they are designed: tennis shoes are getting bouncier and better at absorbing shock; boating shoes are getting better at keeping the feet dry while allowing easy motion in all directions, and so on.

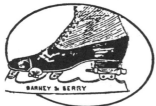

Three factors determine what shoes are right for your sport: the motion it requires of your feet; the surface you will be playing on; and the shape, flexibility, and other idiosyncrasies of your feet and legs. Finding the right shoe, after taking those three factors into consideration, is largely a matter of trial and error. Safety depends on the comfort and fit of your shoes—so keep trying until you find a make and model that works.

We're not going to suggest particular models of shoes here, because they change from season to season as the manufacturers learn more and more from foot specialists about what's best for individual sports. Probably the best source of information about these developments are magazines devoted to individual sports, which usually review new shoe models. Another good source is the salespeople in a good shoe store devoted exclusively to the footwear for your sport.

**RUNNING, JOGGING, AND WALKING** Running shoes, in many ways, are a paradigm of a shoe suited to a sport and to your feet. A runner sets out in one direction—forward—and keeps going the same way. His feet and knees always point forward; his head and body always move straight ahead. Such unidirectional motion is true only of running, walking, jogging, and perhaps jumping rope or weight-lifting; most other sports require movement in several directions. You might leap sideways to catch or hit a ball, or to move backwards to position yourself for a fencing stroke. But with running, an important quality in a shoe is its ability to keep the foot and leg facing securely forward so that you don't twist your knee or ankle, and to cushion your landing well.

The result, in running shoes, is a flared heel, unlike the heels in shoes for other sports. The heel helps control your rear foot and knee as it leaves the ground, keeping the leg's unidirectional movement stable. At the same time, the width of the heel helps absorb the impact of your foot against the ground. This is important, because with each running step you take, your heel may have to endure three to four times the force of your body's weight as it hits the ground. The larger a building's foundations are, the more weight the building can bear; the wider the surface of your heel, the more the shock of landing is dispersed. If our feet continue to evolve in adaptation to concrete surfaces, we may well develop flat heels like those of running shoes, and we'll see far fewer foot and leg injuries occuring from stress. In the meantime, we'll just have to make do with good, flared-heel shoes.

A good running shoe will have to absorb three to four times your weight with each step, again and again. If it doesn't, running will jar and damage the small bones of your feet, or your legs, knees, hips, or spine. So running shoes are made with a special shock-absorbing wedge, called a midsole, inserted between the rubber bottoms and the uppers of the shoe. You can see the sides of this midsole when you look at a good running shoe: it's usually a lighter-colored wedge of material that gives the shoe bottom its added thickness.

The material of these midsoles varies with the shoes. Some are firmer, others emphasize compressibility for improved shock absorption. Which to choose depends on your feet—and your pocketbook. In general, if you have relatively rigid feet, characterized by high arches, you want to aim for maximum flexibility together with high compressibility and shock absorption. If your feet are softer you can usually tolerate a more rigid shoe, since your feet themselves are already somewhat designed for shock absorption.

If you are a big person, you need strong, less flexible running shoes. We know of one doctor who tells heavy football-player types to jog in combat boots rather than running shoes—and he's not far from right. While combat boots don't offer quite enough shock absorption for anyone's long-distance running needs, no matter how large and soft their feet are, such shoes will certainly hold up under the pounding a heavy person is going to give them.

Highly compressible, shock-absorbing midsoles do add spring to the step of someone whose rigid feet might otherwise make running on hard surfaces dangerous to their bones, but this kind of midsole compresses quickly, losing its shock-absorbing value—your shoes may have outlived their usefulness even before the bottom of the sole shows any signs of wear. If you've got rigid, high-arched feet and you want to run—particularly if you want to run long distances—you're going to have to resign yourself, for safety's sake, to spending money on new running shoes frequently so that the shock absorption you need is always there.

In more specific terms: if you're a serious runner, covering ten to twenty miles a day, your running shoes—even if they're the very best—are going to lose their compressibility after a mere six weeks. Perhaps spending forty to sixty dollars every six weeks on a new pair of running shoes sounds like an expensive indulgence, but look at it this way: as a runner, you have very little other equipment to purchase; you can run almost anywhere; and a good, shock-absorbing shoe is the only protection you have. And buying new shoes is a lot less expensive than a visit to the doctor. Giving your feet the protection of a fresh, zippy pair of new running shoes as soon as the old ones lose their bounce is the best insurance you have to keep your feet and legs healthy, to keep running steadily, without having to take time out for shinsplints, stress fractures, and other symptoms of bad shoes or bad alignment.

Of course, if you run shorter distances, your shoes will last longer. While a seventy-five-mile-a-week runner uses up his shoes in about six weeks, if you're a half-an-hour-a-day walker, your shoes may last from six months to a year. And if you walk or run on a dirt track or the grass of a park, they may last you even longer. Just be aware when your shoes have lost their bounce. If you think they have, you're probably right. Then it's time to put them out to pasture—in this case you can save them for foul-weather wear—and invest in a new pair. You'll be delighted at how good and springy they feel on your feet—and at the same time, you'll realize that you'd lost a lot of protection in the old ones. Make a note of how long your old shoes lasted before you retired them. Next time, don't let them reach that point—pick up a new pair *before* the old ones have lost their spring completely. If it's worth it to your health and well-being to run, walk, or jog, it should also be worth it financially to protect your feet and legs with the right shoes.

Running shoes need not cost you an arm and a leg, but it's not a good idea to buy the cheapest you can find, either. Shoes below the forty-dollar range just don't seem to have the combination of protection, flexibility, shock absorption, and comfort that your feet need. On the other hand, unless you have oddly shaped feet that require custom-fitted shoes with special orthopedic devices, there is usually no reason to spend more than forty to sixty dollars (perhaps slightly less if you can find a sale just when you need new shoes) on a pair of running shoes. The very expensive brands, which can cost a hundred dollars and more, do not necessarily afford your feet any more protection—or last any longer—than the moderately-priced shoes.

Unless it has a very unusual sports shoe department, don't try to buy your running shoes at a regular shoestore. Instead, find a good running-wear store that specializes in footgear and equipment, and carries a wide variety of shoes, including the top of the line. That way, you can try on the best shoes and compare them. Another advantage of going to a store that specializes in running gear is that the salespeople will understand your comparison shopping. Most good stores allow you to walk around for a decent period in the shoes you think you like best. At least one store in Manhattan—Super Runner's Shop—lets you jog up and down on the pavement outside for a few minutes to see what the shoes feel like on a concrete surface. Gary Murke, proprietor of that store, and the first winner of the New York Marathon, understands how frustrating it is to buy shoes without knowing whether you will feel good running in them or not.

Although finding the best shoe for your foot is largely a matter of trial and error, there are certain minimal standards we feel a pair of shoes *must* meet:

FIT: Does the shoe conform to the shape of your foot, without pinching your toes, your bunion joint, the tops of your arch, or any other part of your foot? Remember the "rule of thumb": at least a thumbnail's length between your longest toe and the end of the shoe. That's usually at least half an inch—and some people may need a quarter-inch more to make sure their toes don't bump up against the end of the shoe when they run. And don't fall into the trap of thinking that you wear a particular size and *that's it*—in a running shoe, you may need anywhere from a half-size to a size-and-a-half larger than in your street shoes. What counts is not the number, but the actual fit.

But there's more to fit than just the length of the shoe. Take the uppers, for example. Some shoes are cut high in the toe box while others leave little room for your toes. Remember, when you run your toes contract as if to grip the ground, so the joints are slightly raised. If there isn't enough space between your toes and the top of the shoe, with every step you take your joints will graze the nylon surface of the shoe. Before long, this constant irritation may result in corns or other problems, which can call for surgery. If the shoes you're wearing now are comfortable enough in other ways but you've noticed that your joints graze the top of the shoe when you're running, throw them out—they're just not good enough. And as we've said before, the cost of a new pair of shoes doesn't touch the cost of medical care.

Make sure the shoes are wide enough. They shouldn't be pinching your metatarsal joints or your big toe. To test for roominess across the metatarsals—before you buy the shoes—stand up with your weight on the foot you're testing, bend down, and try to get a grip on the material just above your toe joints. You should almost, but not quite, be able to pinch the material up away from the joints. (And of course, if you feel the least bit of pinching, either at your bunion joint or anywhere else, you're wearing the wrong shoes! Running shoes *must* be luxuriously comfortable.) It's important to do this test standing up, since your weight spreads the width of your feet over a larger area—and the force of jogging will make them wider still, with the pressure of each step.

Do you have unusually wide or narrow feet? Unfortunately, only a few companies manufacture running shoes to meet your needs. For very wide feet, try shoes from New Balance of Boston, Van's of California, and Saucony of Massachusetts. If your feet are narrow, see if you can find shoes made by Brook's, New Balance, or Van's.

When you're being fitted—or fitting yourself—for a running shoe, try not to worry too much about the overall appearance or color of the shoe. It is much more important that the shoe combines the proper characteristics for your foot than that it match your running outfit.

COMFORT: Again, if the shoe pinches you, discard it. Most running shoes are now designed with foam-rubber padding that lines the inside of the tongue, and the edge of the upper. The lining keeps your feet from being cut or irritated. In addition, the lace patterns of shoes vary, so choose a shoe that doesn't press on any of the individual bumps and bones of your unique feet when you lace it up. You can ease up on the pressure of the laces at the points at which your feet are boniest. With so many shoes to choose from, you'd be foolish to walk out of a store wondering whether the rubbing you feel on your heel, or the pressure on a bone on the top of your foot, is going to bother you when you walk or run for exercise. You can be sure that it will—and the best way to avoid it is to take those shoes off and go try on another pair until you find the shoe that's comfortable for *you*.

When you get the shoes home, test them again for comfort by wearing them around the house for forty-five minutes to an hour. (You shouldn't wear them longer than that the first time you put them on to break them in, anyway.) If after half-an-hour you find that they hurt your feet just walking around the house, they'll be unbearable when you're running or walking. If the store allows it, take them back and get another pair of shoes. If not, you may just have to face the fact that you've made a rather expensive mistake. Don't compound it by running in ill-fitting shoes that might seriously damage your feet. Cross that shoe model off your list and start your search anew for the shoe that's right for you.

STABILITY AND SUPPORT: Most of today's running shoes combine nylon or other synthetic mesh (for lightness of weight, flexibility, and moisture evaporation), with specially treated leathers that provide stability, support, and control where it is needed in the upper portion of the shoe. When you try the shoes on in the store, make sure that they give you the stability and support you need to run safely and well. And again, make sure that the lacing pattern of the shoes you buy gives you good control and holds the shoe on securely, without rubbing the bumps on your feet.

A final note of warning about running shoes. They are excellent for running, walking, racewalking, jogging, hiking, or any other type of exercise in which you want your feet and knees always to face forward. But *please* don't wear them for tennis, racquetball, squash, jai alai, paddleball, baseball, basketball, or any other sport in which you need to be able to move multidirectionally. If you try to move sideways or swivel around in running shoes, the flared heels can lead to twisted and injured ankles and bones. Just as you wouldn't use a screwdriver to hammer in a nail, don't try to wear running shoes for racquet or field sports. They're just the wrong tool for the job.

**RACQUET SPORTS**   For racquetball, tennis, squash, paddle-ball, and other racquet sports, another factor comes into play in choosing a shoe. Because you want to be able to dart in any direction, twist and turn when necessary, step sideways or diagonally backward, and then pivot to hit the ball or shuttle-cock, you must avoid the flared heel of the running shoe, as it will trip you up dangerously when you try to turn or run sideways. You want a simple shoe that conforms to the shape of your foot and to the terrain on which you will be playing.

If you're just playing badminton on the lawn, your second consideration is a rubber sole and breathable upper material that can wick moisture away from your feet. But for tennis—especially on a concrete court—if you're serious about protection for your feet, legs, and spine, a shock-absorbing, padded sole wouldn't hurt. Unlike in running, when most of your weight comes down on your heels, in racquet sports you've got to be on your toes, so it's the ball of the foot and the toes that take most of the force each time you dash for the ball. Unfortunately, most tennis and racquetball shoes today are not very good for the feet: the soles are thin, with very little compressibility to cushion shock. However, a few manufacturers are starting to adopt a wedge construction that incorporates a layer of shock-absorbing material. If you play often, it wouldn't be a bad idea to look around until you find these more shock-absorbing shoes. The better racquetball shoes also now come with a replaceable shock-absorbing insert.

When you try on your tennis sneakers in a store, the same considerations for fit, comfort, and support apply that we delineated for running shoes. Make sure the toe box is long, high, and wide enough for your toes to have plenty of room to move around, to curl as they grip the ground, and so on. Make sure that the laces keep the shoe on your foot securely, without pinching, and that the seams don't press against bumps in your feet.

If you have very wide or very narrow feet, you may have some difficulty finding shoes that both fit and cushion your feet. At least one company, New Balance, makes very wide widths in racquet sports shoes; New Balance is also the pioneer in developing the more supportive, more compressible styles that other companies are now starting to adopt. (See Appendix C for the addresses of several makers of sports shoes for wide and narrow feet.)

**BASKETBALL**   The traditional basketball sneakers, which many players still prefer, lace all the way up the ankle. But researchers have found that the canvas "high-top" ankle section is too flimsy to give the support that most players really need and can actually restrict motion in some people's ankles, adding to the risk of injury during sudden turns or landings from twist-jumps. For most players, we recommend a regular, low-cut sneaker. You can buy these shoes especially designed for basketball—but in truth, any sneaker designed for multidirectional movement (*not* a running shoe!) will serve your purposes well. The newer tennis and racquetball sneakers with the extra midsole will give you extra shock absorption, which is helpful when you come down from a jump or run across the court.

**BASEBALL**   For baseball, too, normal sneakers will do. Some players, however, because baseball is played outdoors, feel that they play best in a shoe with a soft rubber spike that can dig into the earth, giving them added traction and stability when they run. If you want to wear spiked shoes for playing baseball, that's fine, but remember, never wear shoes with very long, thick spikes or metal-tipped cleats. Wearing long or metal spikes in a sport in which it is not at all uncommon for two players to collide as they are sliding into a base or running to catch a ball is asking for trouble. The protruding cleats, especially if they are metal, can cause serious injury if they inadvertently clip someone in the face, ribs, or skin.

**BOATING**   Boating, rowing, and other sports in which your feet are liable to get wet are best enjoyed in a shoe that allows water to drain away from the sole. Many running shoes, designed to allow perspiration to evaporate, serve this function. Running shoes are just fine if you are rowing or just sitting in a deck chair enjoying the scenery. But if you're actively involved in sailing or steering a boat as it weaves through the waves, running shoes may not be the best choice. They *will* help keep your feet dry—and therefore prevent the soles from getting too slippery—but those flared heels can cause ankle or knee trouble when you've got to jump sideways or turn around fast as the boat rocks. Some of the newer boating or deck shoes are designed both to wick water away from the soles of the feet and to allow multidirectional freedom of motion. These may be ideal. But tennis sneakers made of light nylon might suit your needs just as well.

**ROLLER SKATING**    Roller skate boots are designed with the primary requirements of the skater in mind: balance and the ability to shift weight evenly from one edge of the boot to the other, in order to steer and turn. What's needed here is a rigid leg, so that the ankle won't wobble and distort the shifts in weight. Needless to say, weak, wobbly ankles can lead not just to poor skating, but to a high risk of injury to ankles, knees, and any other part of your body that might be jarred or scraped in a fall.

The most important part of the skate boot, therefore, is the counter—the rigid piece of material that runs up the back of the ankle from the heel, as well as midway down the sides of the heel. It is designed to support the ankle in place, which it just can't do if the material is broken down or worn out. If that's the case, replace your skates.

Because roller skating is an exhibition sport, many skates are designed to look fashionable, with narrow, pointed toes. When you shop for skates, please don't sacrifice comfort for appearance. As with any other shoe, your skate boot should fit properly, with the right toe length, width, and height for comfort. The fit in the toe box is especially important, because the toe box is so rigid that you certainly don't want your toes banging up against it.

If you're using your skates for special or trick skating, or for disco dancing, you'll need some extra shock absorption (though not so much as to mar your ability to transmit subtle degrees of pressure to the wheel edges). Invest in some shock-absorbing insoles made especially for roller skates.

Make sure that the lace pattern of your skates fits your feet comfortably. Don't tie them so tightly that you restrict your circulation, or so loosely that you lose ankle stability. And every so often while you're skating, stop to adjust your laces, as long shoelaces tend to loosen and shift as you move. (By the way, this is good advice for all sports activities.)

**CYCLING** We've been asked many times whether a special cycling shoe is really necessary. Although these are popular with some serious cyclists, our answer is still "no." The advantage of a cycling shoe is that it fits well into the toeclips which should always be on the pedals to keep your feet from slipping off, and it does transfer force more readily to the pedals as you cycle. But really, any flat-bottomed shoe will do—tennis or racquetball sneakers, basketball or baseball shoes—unless, of course, you are a serious competitive cyclist. You can even wear your running shoes: the flared heel won't hurt your ankles or knees, since there is no sideways motion involved in pedaling. But one thing to consider here is that, in cycling, force is transmitted through the forefoot, not through the heel, as in running. So a shoe with extra forefoot—rather than heel—shock absorption will be more comfortable.

As with any other shoe, make sure that whatever footwear you use for cycling has adequate toe room—front, side, and top—and that your bunion joint is not squeezed. When you ride, you should also make sure that the toeclips are on firmly, but not too tight. Toeclips can squeeze an already-tight shoe, which will make your feet really uncomfortable. Not only must your shoe fit, but your toe clips must also fit over it properly. Another bit of advice: never ride your bicycle without toeclips on the pedals, which prevent accidental slips of the foot as well as increasing efficiency and working more of your leg muscles.

**GOLF** The metal cleats of golf shoes don't carry the same risks as hard baseball cleats, because the game doesn't involve much possibility of bumping into someone else with your feet. They do, however, pose some risks to the wearer: be careful, when walking between shots, not to get caught in potholes where you can twist an ankle if the cleats catch too deeply. The purpose of cleats in golf is not for efficient walking, but for traction and stability when you're swinging the club: they grip the ground to help you keep your feet planted firmly. One way to help your golf shoes help you in your swinging action is to clean out the mud between the cleats between swings, so that they won't slip and trip you up.

As an alternative to golf shoes, you can wear almost any rubber-soled athletic shoe. Don't wear normal, leather-soled street shoes, which will be too slippery for the green, or running shoes, as the flared heels can limit rotary movement of the ankles and knees.

**WEIGHT LIFTING**   There are special boots for weight lifting, but a flat-soled running shoe is perhaps an even better choice of footgear. By flat-soled, we mean not nubbed on the bottom. It's fairly easy to find a running shoe that just has small lines or ridges running along the bottom of the shoe, and that's what you're looking for. If you're lifting weights, this shoe will give you shock absorbability as well as medial and lateral stability. The point is, you're not going anywhere, and you certainly don't want your feet to slide out from under you while you're standing there under a weight. The wide, flared heel of a running shoe will cushion your foot, at the same time keeping your knees and ankles straight ahead, as they should be, while the flat soles enable you to keep your feet firmly on the floor.

**WRESTLING AND BOXING**   If you compete in either of these martial arts, you know that for competition specially designed leather boots—which usually have a suede sole, are fairly lightweight, and let you move quickly from side to side or in any other direction—are required. Since these boots don't give you much shock absorption, you may want to add a shock-absorbing insole. If you plan to do that, plan *ahead* by buying a boot that leaves room for the insole insert in the bottom. In other words, make sure that the toe box is wide and high enough so that you can add a bit of height without having your toes scrape the top of the boot.

For practice, almost any multidirectional athletic shoe will do. Running shoes are out, since they hamper sideways motion.

**FENCING** Traditionally, fencers wear demi-boots with leather insoles—footgear which is flexible, allowing your foot to slide easily along the floor when necessary, or to grip it when you're standing your ground. Their disadvantage is their limited shock absorption. As a shock-absorbing alternative, you might try wearing a flat-soled, multidirectional athletic shoe, like a tennis or racquetball shoe. Better yet, simply insert a shock-absorbing insole into your fencing boot. Of course, this means that your boot must be big enough to accommodate the extra insole. Check when buying the boots that you have adequate toe room not only in height but in width and length, so that you won't bruise or irritate your feet as you move along the floor in a too-tight boot.

## SOCKS FOR SPORTS

It may sound silly, but the socks you're wearing can make all the difference between enjoying yourself and playing your best, whatever your sport, and being uncomfortable, cranky, and off your game. Since you want to play your best—even if you're not competing, but merely running, skiing, or volleying for the sheer joy of exercise and play—you'll find that it's worthwhile to pay attention to certain items usually thought of as insignificant—like socks.

The primary purpose of socks is to keep your feet comfortable and as dry as possible inside your shoes. (Complementing the color and line of your sportswear is, hopefully, by far a secondary consideration.) Socks that are too tight will bind your feet. Socks that are too large may bunch up, causing blisters, skin irritations, pain, and calluses. The wrong socks can make you uncomfortable and distracted while you're playing, so take the time while you're shopping for socks to make sure you're buying good socks that *fit*.

The best socks for most sports are made of cotton, or cotton and Orlon. These materials are good because they act like the wick of a candle, drawing perspiration up and away from your feet, leaving them relatively dry and sweet-smelling while you work up a sweat. Synthetics, especially nylon, do the opposite: they insulate your feet, leaving them sticky, sweaty, hot, and most likely smelly, too. And smelly feet are not something you want to avoid just to please your neighbors in the locker room. Smelly feet are an almost sure sign that large numbers of microorganisms are breeding on the surfaces and in the warm, moist crevices of your skin. If your skin is at all sensitive to any of these flora and fauna, you're inviting athlete's foot or some other kind of fungus infection, like fungus nails. The best prevention is just not to wear nylon or any other synthetic in the belly of your socks. (If you like a little nylon elastic to hold your socks up at the ankles, that's a completely different matter, and quite all right.)

In winter, for sports such as ice skating, skiing, and hockey, you will want the warmth of wool for your feet, but you also need something with the ability of cotton to wick away perspiration. The best solution for this dual need is to wear two pairs of socks: a thin undersock of cotton, and a warm outer sock of wool to keep out the cold.

For the rest of the year, a medium-thick cotton sock is your best bet. Wear regular socks for spring and fall, anklets—if you prefer—for summer, and knee socks for winter. The best color for socks year-round is white, although this choice is bound to offend the aesthetic sensibility of more than a few people. Why white? Especially if your feet perspire a lot, and even more especially if your skin is sensitive to chemicals, you should avoid colored socks, which contain synthetic dyes. If your sweat mixes with and dissolves the dye from your socks, you may not only find that your skin is tinged with the color of the socks, but that it itches and smarts, too.

Dyes are not the only chemicals found in socks. Some athletic socks are advertised as combatting foot odor. Good hygiene is the best way to prevent foot odor; beyond that, some people are going to react to the odor-killing chemicals more severely than they would to the microorganisms that cause the smell in the first place.

We can't say it too often: Change your socks at least once every day. If you perspire a lot, change whenever your socks get wet to prevent the warm, moist environment in which fungus thrives. Whatever you do, *never* wear a pair of socks twice in a row without having washed them: fungus and bacteria grow at an alarming rate in sweaty socks, and wearing yesterday's socks can only lead to tomorrow's sensitivity reactions or infections.

If you're concerned that your socks will wear out too fast if you keep changing them and putting them in the wash, just don't do it! As long as they aren't actually dirty, but merely sweaty, your socks can be cleaned by soaking them in a sink filled with warm water. Change the water every ten or fifteen minutes for half an hour or longer, and let them drip dry overnight. This prevents the fibers and elastic in the socks from being prematurely worn out by soaps, detergents, or the heat of the washer and dryer. And of course, it will also protect your skin from the harsh effects of soap or detergent residue that might otherwise remain in your socks. Of course, hand-washing takes a little more time than throwing your dirty socks in the hamper, but buying new socks is time-consuming, too.

## ORTHOTIC DEVICES

The body is a unit, one organism, composed of parts designed to help you walk properly; any "tunnel vision" approach to foot and leg problem that *keeps* you from walking properly just won't work here. All the parts of your body that are involved in walking have to be in a healthy state, in the correct functional position, for you to walk properly and with ease. If one of the body parts you need to walk is out of position or unhealthy you're not going to be able to walk as well, and may even suffer pain. A house that is unlevel at the foundation will not only develop problems in the basement, but the walls may start cracking even on the top floors. By the same token, if part of your foot, leg, or thigh is out of position, you may suffer low back and hip trouble, groin troubles, sciatica, neck stiffness, and upper back problems.

In the past, a great many foot and leg problems were routinely attributed to the arches. If the arches were low, orthopedists almost automatically assumed that the feet were "bad." If the arches were high, that was "good." We now know not only that a high arch actually presents more of a potential problem than a low one, but also that most leg and foot imbalances aren't the arches' fault at all.

Factors that more often cause imbalances are improper time sequences in the way the foot and leg move when you walk, and hereditary factors. A proper time sequence for your foot and leg can be developed with the help of an orthopedist or a physical therapist, or by using an orthotic device; hereditary factors may present more of a difficulty, and vary widely in seriousness. A mild structural imbalance inherited from your parents or grandparents may not show up as a problem until you yourself are in your sixties, seventies, or eighties, when you may blame it on a pair of new shoes or old age. But a severe orthopedic imbalance may be obvious as early as childhood, especially in an active child.

Some inherited problems manifest themselves earlier if you wear improper footgear, don't exercise properly, or perform work that puts stress on your legs and feet. In a sense, you are fortunate if your inherited imbalance rears its head early; if you are aware of it you can treat it properly. While braces and arch supports used to be the most-often prescribed treatments for imbalances, we now know the *orthotic device* to be most effective. An orthotic device may look like an arch support to the untrained eye, but it is really more than that. A timing device for the foot and leg, the orthotic device holds the bone structure of the foot in its ideal position, allowing the proper stress to pass through each bone and joint at just the right moment. It forces bones to do their fair share of the work in bearing weight and stress, and causes muscles to pull at the right angles, at the right time.

In turn, the stress that travels up through the leg and into the hip and lower back is dissipated in a natural way. This prevents buildup of stress in certain key areas—the knees, the hips, or the lower back—which can cause weakness and injury. About ninety percent of ankle, knee, hip, and lower-back trouble can be controlled with an orthotic device, in fact, if the trouble stems from a structural imbalance in the first place. Yet, oddly enough, orthotics are only about seventy-five percent effective in controlling foot trouble.

Before orthotic devices, or even arch supports, were invented, a common way of dealing with a foot or leg imbalance was with specially made shoes. However, even the tightest-laced shoe, with corrections made on the soles or heels with wedges, allows the foot to move around *inside* the shoe, which means that the structural problem is not addressed properly. Specially made shoes were also used to "correct" children's feet when bones were out of position at birth: if the metatarsal bone was twisted in, for example, a shoe would actually twist the foot back toward the outside. We now know that such therapy wreaks havoc with many of the joints inside the foot, and doctors have stopped using it for the most part.

Devices such as arch cookies—simple foam cushions covered by leather and worn in the bottom of the shoes—break down completely when the foot pronates (twists in at the ankle), and do not really control the *structure* of the foot at all. One of the few such devices that does seem to help is a rubber metatarsal raise, which eases pain in the metatarsal joints. These simple, inexpensive lifts can raise flexible metatarsals closer to a normal level, reducing the pressure and controlling discomfort; but they cannot stop further dropping of the metatarsal bone as a good orthotic device would do, and are thus only a stopgap.

If you have a mild foot imbalance, a homemade orthotic device may help. Pieces of leather or cotton felt, in half-, quarter-, or even eighth-inch thicknesses, can be layered within the shoe to fill in the arch area on the inside of the foot, "neutralizing" the position of the ankle joint so it neither twists in, nor twists out. The materials needed are inexpensive, and available in most surgical supply stores.

In the past few years, storebought orthotics, beneficial in controlling the mildly imbalanced foot structure, have become very popular. Dr. Scholl's runner's wedge is an excellent device even for a walker. When purchasing a storebought orthotic device, whether from a drugstore or from a shoe-store, it is important to discriminate between genuine orthotic devices and arch supports. The latter are not, in general, truly beneficial. A storebought orthotic, can be customized for your foot with layers of leather or felt, as we discussed above, and can actually help to rebalance the foot structure. More serious problems of foot imbalance require professionally made orthotics, available from podiatrists, chiropractors, and orthopedic surgeons, and tailor-made from a cast of your foot.

Whether you are using a homemade, storebought, or professionally made orthotic device, remember to break it in slowly. Ligaments and muscles in your feet and legs have been tightened and shortened, while others have been stretched and overused. These imbalances have to right themselves slowly and steadily in order to stabilize at their natural equilibrium. So no matter how comfortable the orthotic device feels—and if it's the right one, it may feel very comfortable indeed—let your foot adjust to it gradually.

Just about the only type of orthotic device that works in dress shoes, ski boots, ice or roller skating boots, ballet shoes, pumps, and boots—in general, all the wrong shoes for your feet—is a new device called a halfdotic. Made by Langer Biomechanics (see Appendix C) in a cobra pattern, this device is extremely thin and simple, yet gives a good deal of control to the foot structure. Of course, the halfdotics are not nearly as effective as a full orthotic, but if you have a serious imbalance it's important to wear the halfdotic when you're wearing the "wrong" shoes, and a full orthdotic the rest of the time.

FLAT-FOOTEDNESS is one very common condition that may be relieved by an orthodic device. As we said earlier, flat feet were once blamed for most structural imbalances. We now know the folly of that reasoning, but flat-footed people may indeed feel less discomfort if they use an orthodic device, particularly if they walk and stand a lot.

HIGH-ARCHED FEET, the most rigid type of feet, really do not need an orthodic device, though they can benefit from shock absorption. Running shoes are great for protecting the foot, cushioning it against the stress of walking on hard surfaces. You can also purchase shock-absorbing insoles that will do the trick, such as PPT from Langer Biomechanics, Spenco, and Sorbathane II. Most of these can be purchased in a store, although there is now also a Sorbathane II medical-grade insole that is sold only through doctors' offices. Try to choose an insole that is neither too heavy nor too bulky for your foot—comfort, after all, is just as important as protection.

BUNIONS, HAMMER TOES, AND HEEL ABNORMALITIES—often hereditary conditions, caused by bones moving out of position—may also call for help from orthotic devices. They don't usually show up in childhood, but develop slowly from sheer wear and tear. Stress and activity can accelerate the development of any of these conditions. Hammer toes and bunions are best controlled with the use of professional orthotic devices, the kind your podiatrist or doctor prescribes for you. Hammer toes can also be helped by simple stretching of the toes, as well as orthotic control and proper foot gear. Bunions, although less easily corrected, can be prevented completely from forming simply by using the proper orthodic device and wearing the right shoes. If you have either bunions or hammer toes and don't take measures to control or correct them, you may find yourself with medical problems that are far more costly and difficult to treat.

Remember, an uncorrected foot and leg imbalance can lead to lower back, hip, and upper back problems. If you have pain in any of these areas and are not being helped by the therapy your doctor has prescribed, you might see an orthopedist to determine if the problem can be traced to your feet and legs.

**ORTHOTIC DEVICES FOR CHILDREN**  Children are sometimes born with certain structural problems that call for the help of an orthopedist even before they're walking. In-toe and out-toe problems, discussed in Chapter 1, are examples of such conditions. As you may remember, most babies are born with their thigh bones twisted *out*. If the thigh bones twist in, they should be corrected immediately. While some doctors advocate putting the legs in a cast, in our 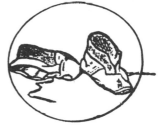 opinion this is one of the worst methods for treating either out-toeing or in-toeing. Casting causes atrophy of muscles, which results in a natural weakening effect, loss of bone minerals, and even development of arthritic joints. We feel that the long-term effects of casting infants have not been properly studied. In most cases the condition can be just as easily corrected with proper exercise, which stretches the muscles, and therefore the bone cartilage, of the legs. (By exercise here we mean manipulation of the infant's legs by the parents or doctor.) In more severe cases, special types of splints can be prescribed for the baby to wear while it is asleep. In even more severe cases, the splints might also be worn in the daytime before the child begins walking. Recently, Langer Biomechanics has developed a revolutionary device, sometimes called the "nightbar," to help correct this problem after the child has started walking. It attaches to the child's shoe, allowing him to walk and crawl while wearing it, and is easily removable for diaper-changes or whatever—so as well as being a good corrective device, it is also a real time-saver.

By the time a child is two or three, the thigh bone should not be as fully rotated out as it was when she was born, or out-toeing will be a problem. Many doctors tell parents that out-toeing will correct itself by early adolescence. However, sometimes that is not the case, which presents real problems at age twelve or thirteen. Fortunately, out-toeing can be corrected in a young child with the same device that we just described for controlling in-toeing, adjusted accordingly.

If a child refuses to wear the nightbar, out-toeing and in-toeing can also be corrected by orthotics that actually force the foot to twist in or out, as the case may be, with each step the child takes. While this method must be used over a much longer period of time, it is worth it for the results it usually brings.

There is one case in which casting may be necessary: children who are born with a clubfoot. These children have their feet twisted to the outside so severely that they could end up walking on their outside ankle bones and the sides of their feet, rather than their soles. This congenital abnormality is generally immediately obvious to a doctor, and treated shortly after the child is born. But if you suspect that your baby's feet are not in a normal position and that your pediatrician has failed to notice it, be sure to bring it up with him or her, and then perhaps consult an orthopedist as well. This type of problem is serious, requiring serial casting techniques (several stages of casting), as well as physical therapy, in some cases. And the sooner you catch the problem the better; a baby's feet are highly malleable, since they are mainly cartilage, without many fully developed muscles, ligaments, and tendons yet. The right kind of therapy, used early enough, can implement a tremendous and fairly painless change.

Knock-knees and bowlegs can also be a problem in children. Knock-knees are often related to in-toeing, and bowlegs to out-toeing, though mineral deficiencies can also be responsible for either problem. Through certain stages of your child's life, knock-knees and bowlegs can be normal, but it's still best to consult with a podiatrist, orthopedic surgeon, or physician to see if therapy is needed. If therapy is suggested, get second and third opinions as to the right course of action. Knock-knees and bowlegs rarely, if ever, need casting; they are usually best corrected through exercise therapy and the use of the proper orthotic device.

# MASSAGE

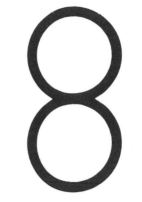

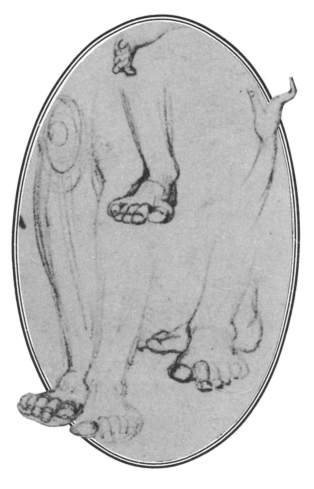

MASSAGE—OFTEN WITH medicinal herbs and oils—has been used to help heal muscular injuries, sprains, and strains for centuries. Early civilization's healers found that massage not only promoted healing but might even save lives; a person unable to escape danger because of a physical disability did not stay alive very long. Our lives may rarely depend on massage now, but without it stress and injuries may unnecessarily limit our productivity.

Almost every culture has developed some form of massage. In past centuries massage was often available only to the wealthy or the military class, however—rarely could the common man afford such luxury. Today, massage is within everyone's reach. Forms of massage developed independently in widely-differing cultures—swedish massage and Japanese shiatsu, to name two—are used around the world and combined with each other to create new methods. The varying styles of massage are similar in philosophy and in the desired goals; often most effective is the combination of two or more massage techniques, enhancing each other in the same therapy session. Therapists who use only one technique are self-limited.

135

## BENEFITS OF MASSAGE

Massage can be used to treat injuries caused by work, athletics, and accidents. It reduces the tension which causes back pain, muscular tenderness and tightness, headaches, swelling in the legs and feet, and weakening of the immune system. Regular massage, one to three times a week, can help prevent 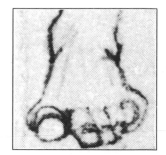 as well as safely treat these problems, as well as reduce the strains of athletic performance.

To understand how massage can accomplish so many wonderful things we must first understand what happens when our muscles or tendons are injured or caused to overtighten. First the muscle and tendon fibers contract; they become brittle and inelastic, easy to tear. This tightness causes electrochemical changes in the salts found within and outside each muscle-tendon cell; as a result, fluid gathers around the cells, and trapped protein molecules cluster and bind together. Thus, a swelling forms around the cells, made up of lymph (body fluid) and protein molecules, and the return flow of lymph through the lymphotic circulatory system is blocked. This disruption in lymph flow puts pressure on the nerve endings in and around the muscle-tendon cells, and cause pain in the muscle.

Massage reverses this process. First, it breaks up the clusters of protein cells that block the flow of lymph fluid out of the muscle-tendon fibers. Electrochemical balance is restored; finally, the muscle-tendon fibers relax. When these fibers are relaxed, energy is consumed and utilized more effectively. High blood pressure caused by constriction of arteries from tight muscles is often reduced. The circulation to injured cells returns to normal, bringing in nutrients and removing toxins and waste products. As muscles relax, tension and anxiety are reduced. This can help prevent injuries, headaches, muscular aches and, very importantly, depression and all its consequences.

By now you probably are wondering why apparently so few people have availed themselves of this wonderful healing and energy-enhancing therapy. The answer may be found in our increasingly complex society, where simple and beneficial methods of healing are often overlooked in favor of more complex, frequently dangerous or toxic, methods. Modern traditional medicine thrives on complexity and toxicity, choosing to overlook or minimize the benefits of older, proven healing methods.

Try self-massage or, even better, have someone you love give you a massage. Frequently, people will say that they don't know how to give a good massage—but *any* massage is good. Just do what feels natural and pleasing. There *are* some basic principles and techniques that will help you get the most out of massage, though. In the following sections we will guide you through two different massage routines. The first, designed to take from six to ten minutes, is easy to do by yourself. It is ideal as a wake-up tonic for your feet and legs in the morning, or to soothe them after a hard day. The second, more in-depth massage will take between thirty minutes and an hour; it is best administered by a friend, and is meant for maximal therapeutic benefit.

## THE TEN-MINUTE MORNING MASSAGE

The best preparation for any foot massage is relaxation. Take a nice hot bath to relax your muscles or—if you don't have time for that—just lie down on the floor, close your eyes, and "let yourself go" by taking long, slow, deep breaths for three to five minutes. Then 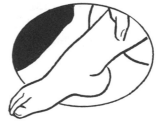 open your eyes very slowly—if you let the light hit your retinas suddenly, your muscles will contract and your relaxation will have been in vain. In fact, take at least two minutes to open your eyes.

Now that you're relaxed, you can start the foot massage. It helps to have baby powder or an oil like sunflower, safflower, or soy oil—which moisturizes the skin at the same time—on hand. If you are fortunate enough to have someone massage your foot and leg, the best position to be in is lying on your back. If you must do it yourself, sit up with your back supported against a wall or firm chair. This will prevent back strain. Start at the toes and work your way back to the heel and then on up the leg. First, manipulate all of the joints in your toes. Flex them one at a time in each of the toes—the metatarsal joints, the bunion joints, and the ones further back. Then flex the ankle joint by rotating your foot in a circle to loosen the whole area up.

The best way to rotate your foot is to cross your legs, hold the leg of the crossed leg just above the ankle bones, and relax the foot completely. The point here is *not* to use the muscles of your foot to rotate it—that wouldn't be very relaxing—but to use your hands, and let your foot just flop. Just take the front portion of your foot and slowly turn the whole thing in small, slow circles. Go first in one direction, then in the other; alternate directions for at least a minute. This loosens up and lubricates your ankle joint with synovial fluid, a clear liquid manufactured in our joints to lubricate the cartilage. Synovial fluid also softens your ligaments—those panels of tissue that make your joints stable—and keeps them pliable, so getting the fluid into the joints on a regular basis is a good way to prevent sprains. As we age, the natural production of synovial fluid lessens, making it especially important to warm up and lubricate the joints.

After you've rotated each foot for about a minute, gently massage the musculature of each foot, top and bottom. You can use your fingertips to knead the feet with varying amounts of pressure. Move them in circles. You can also use the heels of your hands, or your whole hand, to gently squeeze and knead the muscles and flesh. Don't be afraid to use pressure, unless you are very sensitive to it. In that case, you can just lightly rub your feet.

Massage should start with the toes and work all the way up the leg, to the thigh. To do it properly, spend at least three to five minutes on each leg. That may seem like a long time, but it's really not so very much time and effort to put into preventing injury to your feet and legs by keeping them pliable, which is what you're doing. (If you use an oil, you are also giving them a great moisturizing treatment!)

## IN-DEPTH FOOT AND LEG MASSAGE

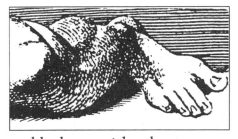

A complete massage of the legs and feet will take between fifteen and thirty minutes per side. Put aside the time. Why rush such a pleasant and energizing experience? Missing any section of tissue or point of energy blockage with a hasty massage may minimize the positive effects of the entire massage. So take your time and focus on what you are experiencing. Always be in touch with your body's sensations, and communicate them to the person massaging you. This will allow them to concentrate the massage on areas and points that need it most, for maximal benefit.

A quiet room with dim lighting will be most relaxing. A noisy, bright room will work against the stress-reducing benefits of the massage. However, massage feels great and will benefit you wherever you can get it. The room temperature should be warm enough to prevent a chill. While scented massage oils are generally available in health stores, cold-pressed safflower or sunflower oil is less costly and will usually work as well. You may add your own fragrance if you wish. Avoid powders for massage; they are unhealthy to breathe into the lungs. Remember to protect the floor, mat, bed, or massage table from the oil with sheets or towels.

Massage is best performed in five simple stages. Stage I is performed with short-fast-light strokes. Stage II is characterized by long, firm strokes. Stage III is a form of acupressure, like shiatsu, which works on energy points. Stage IV is accomplished by firm fast pressure *across* the muscle and tendon fibers. Finally, Stage V is a repeat of the first stage, with short-fast-light strokes. In each stage, begin with the tip of the toes and work up. This will encourage proper lymph circulation and energy flow. Never start with the legs and work toward the toes as this can block lymph and energy flow.

All five stages have equal importance. While each stage we will describe seems slightly more important than the one preceding it, all have equal importance. Each enhances the preceding stage, and brings with it a new benefit, the sum total of which maximize the healing effects of the massage.

STAGE I breaks up swelling in the muscles and tendons and encourages fluids to flow out of the muscle fibers and into the lymph channels (pathways). This is accomplished by a short-fast-light stroking of the fibers towards the heart. When muscle fibers are sore, or tender this stroke may hurt slightly. After only twenty to thirty seconds, however, the discomfort will usually diminish—remember, much of the pain is caused by trapped fluid between the muscle cells. This stroke should be repeated for up to one minute along the entire length of the muscle. Begin at the bottom of the foot and work back towards the heel. Next go to the top of the foot and work from the toes to the ankle. Continue this process from the ankle to the knee both in front and in back of the lower leg. Next work from the knee gradually to the hip. This process directs the flow of extra lymph fluid towards the major collection area in the groin. If a particular area hurts more to the touch spend more time on it, but always be very gentle.

STAGE II uses very firm, long, slow strokes. As in Stage I, begin at the toes and stroke first towards the ankle, both on top and bottom of the feet. Next stroke from the ankle to the knee and finally from the knee to hip. Use the palm of your hand and the area between your thumb and index finger. It is very important to add more and more pressure with each stroke to help force out the extra fluid from the muscle fibers. If a particular area is very painful, go back to Stage I for that area before continuing. At this stage lotions or creams will allow the hand to slide easily over the skin—if no lubricant is used the skin may begin to feel tender and irritated. The smooth sliding action is important to help relax the muscle fibers and can help reduce anxiety and general tension. This stage may take from five to fifteen minutes per leg to complete.

STAGE III requires slow careful pressure applied to each point on the foot and leg, beginning at the toes and again working towards the hip. You may use your thumbs, your fingertips, or both. Press down gently and feel for a firm, small lump of tissue (often the size of a pea) under the skin, deep in the muscle or tendon, as 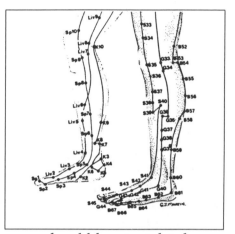 well as around them. The pressure should be straight down. These points follow the patterns of acupuncture points called meridians. Not all the places along these lines will be painful. If there is no pain or discomfort, move to the next place on the skin. As you come closer to active points, discomfort will mount, often changing to pain when you are over an active point. It is important to breathe deeply; shallow breathing blocks lymph flow, while deep breaths pump fluids up to the center of the chest as well as reducing the pain the acupressure may cause.

Press for ten to thirty seconds over each very painful point. Press only one or two seconds over non-painful points. Press each painful point three times, trying to go deeper each time. Picture each painful, firm spot as a balloon that you are trying to "pop." When the point is broken it will no longer feel firm, though it may still feel painful to the touch. People are often surprised to feel these active points as they had no idea that they were there.

Charts are not necessary—discomfort and pain will lead you to the correct places as geiger counters lead to radioactive material. The vast majority of points will be found on the bottom of the feet, including the toes, as well as on the calf and the rear thigh. Few exist on the top of the foot and the front of the leg, so don't waste too much time there. Working the entire bottom of the foot will catch any and all reflexology points, which are known to help many problems in the upper body. Reflexology points are the acupuncture points in the foot that affect parts of our upper body and internal organs.

STAGE IV is performed by rubbing transversely—*across* the muscle or tendon fibers—with very fast, short strokes. Increase the pressure gradually. This stroke can help break up adhesions, a form of internal scar tissue on an injured or overused muscle or tendon. Breaking up adhesions returns normal elasticity and a normal range of motion to the muscle or tendon. Spend more time over the most painful areas or points, using your fingertips as well as the palm of your hand there. The time it takes to complete this stage varies depending on individual need. Begin with the toes and work your way up to the hip.

The amount of time spent massaging your feet and legs is determined by several factors. If your muscles are tight, injured or lack adequate blood circulation for any reason, more time should be devoted to massage. How much time will be determined by such factors as who is massaging you; how much free time you have available; the cost if done professionally (they charge by the hour usually); and the patience, perserverence, and fatigue of the massager, to name a few. A maximal theraputic effect is probably obtained somewhere between fifteen and thirty minutes per foot and leg in most people.

STAGE V repeats Stage I, completing the "circle of massage" therapy. This stage may be repeated during the day as frequently as every fifteen minutes.

# Appendix A:
# AN ANATOMICAL
# FRAMEWORK

## THE SKELETAL SYSTEM

BONES SUPPORT THE body and give it shape, as well as providing a framework for muscle attachments and allowing movement through the joints. Most of us think of bones as the lifeless hard objects we remember from science class skeletons, but in fact bone is alive, and constantly rebuilding itself. New bone cells replace old, dead ones; blood vessels bring in nutrients and remove waste products within the bones just as they do in other body tissues.

Growing bone, however, is found only in children. The bones of the foot and leg usually stop growing by the age of sixteen for girls and seventeen for boys. In infants most of the bone is actually soft, moldable, developing tissue called *cartilage*. In adults cartilage is mostly found lining the joints, where it allows for fluid movements and prevents the bones from grinding at the joints.

A brief tour of the bones of the foot and leg would start at the pelvis. The *pelvic girdle*, which supports the trunk and provides attachment for the leg bones, is actually three bones, the *ilium* at the top and the *ischium* and *pubis* below it, which fuse together in the adult. The thigh bone, or *femur*, fits into a deep socket called the *acetabulum*, at the point where all three parts of the pelvis meet. The femur is the longest and heaviest bone of the body. At the knee it joins the tops of the two lower leg bones, the *tibia* and the *fibula*. The kneecap, or *patella*,

# Anatomy of the Foot and Leg

**ARTERIES AND VEINS
OF THE LOWER LIMB**

Femoral a.

Long saphenous v.

Popliteal a.

Ant. tibial a.

Post. tibial a.

Ant. tibial a.

SUPERFICIAL
VEINS

Med. planter a.

Lat. planter a.

Dorsal pedis a.

**PELVIS
(post. aspect)**

Ilium
Ischium
Pubis
Acetabulum

**TYPICAL JOINT**

Synovial fluid
Periosteum
Cartilage
Synovial
membrane
Bone

Navicular
Tibia
Cuneiform
Talus
Metatarsal
Tarsal
Calcaneus
Cuboid
**MEDIAL ARCH**
Phalanges

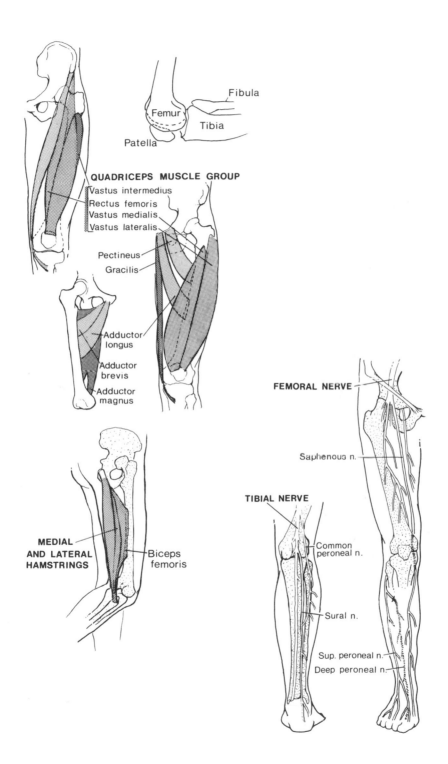

Fibula

Femur

Tibia

Patella

**QUADRICEPS MUSCLE GROUP**

Vastus intermedius
Rectus femoris
Vastus medialis
Vastus lateralis

Pectineus

Gracilis

Adductor longus

Adductor brevis

Adductor magnus

**MEDIAL AND LATERAL HAMSTRINGS**

Biceps femoris

**FEMORAL NERVE**

Saphenous n.

**TIBIAL NERVE**

Common peroneal n.

Sural n.

Sup. peroneal n.

Deep peroneal n.

articulates with the femur but is not actually attached to the bones of the lower leg; it "floats," suspended by the tendons of the muscles at the front of the thigh. It is movable, and helps to increase the leverage of muscles used to straighten the knee. The tibia and fibula end at the ankle joint. The tibia, which is the larger of the two, articulates with the foot to form the ankle joint; it also forms the inner ankle bone.

Each foot has twenty-six bones! These can be divided into the *tarsal* bones—equivalent to the wrist of the hand—the *metatarsal* bones, and the *phalanges*, or toe bones. The *talus* is the uppermost ankle bone, which articulates with the tibia; below and behind it is the *calcaneus*, or heel bone. Further forward are two bones called the *navicular*, on the inside, and the *cuboid*, on the outside. Three bones called the *cuneiforms* form a link between the navicular and the three inside metatarsal bones. The five long *metatarsal* bones run along the top of the foot to the toes, and correspond to the bones of the back of the hands. The metatarsal joints correspond to the knuckles of the hand. Each toe has three bones—the *phalanges*—except the big toe, which has only two. Underneath the bunion joint are two round bones, called *accessory bones*, which help when we step forward. Many people have extra small accessory bones, which can be found near any of the bones of the foot.

The bones of the foot are arranged into two longitudinal arches to bear weight while standing and provide leverage while walking. The *medial arch* of the foot, on the inside, contains the calcaneus, talus, navicular, cuneiform, and the first three metatarsals; its "keystone" is the navicular, and it rests on the calcaneus at the back and the metatarsals at the front. The outside, shallower arch consists of the calcaneus, cuboid, and two outside metatarsals; its keystone is the cuboid. Flat-footedness results when these arches are unusually shallow; it can either be inherited, in the structure of the bones themselves, or result from muscle weakness.

## THE STRUCTURE OF JOINTS

At the joints, the places where two bones meet, *cartilage*—a tough, elastic tissue—covers the ends of the bones, acting as a shock absorber and preventing the bones from grinding together. A membrane known as the *synovial membrane* forms a capsule around the joint. The synovial membrane produces *synovial fluid*, a slippery liquid which fills the space inside the capsule, around and between the bones. As well as lubricating the joint for easy movement, the synovial fluid nourishes the cartilage, which contains no blood vessels. The tissue that lines the cartilage is called the *perichondrium*; the lining of the joint itself is the *periosteum*.

*Ligaments*, thick, fibrous bands of tissue of various lengths, attach around all joints, and sometimes within joints, to keep them stable. They allow the joint to move only within its normal range and proper directions. By aligning the joints correctly they enable muscles and tendons to work efficiently and prevent excessive wear and tear on the joints. *Tendons*, thin, shiny, extremely strong bands of fibrous tissue, make up the link between muscles and bones. Tendons are similar to ligaments, except that they connect muscles to bones rather than bones to each other. Among the muscles, bones, tendons and ligaments around a joint, fluid-filled sacs called *bursae* are distributed, which help to keep all of these structures moving easily against each other.

## THE MUSCLES

MUSCLES work in groups to allow complex series of movements such as walking to take place. Muscle contractions cause the tendons to exert a force where they are attached to the bone and pull it toward them. Muscles have their own circulation and nerve supply. Cut the nerves and muscles stop working; decrease circulation and they fatigue quickly.

The front of the thigh is composed of four main muscles—the *rectus femoris*, the *vastus lateralis*, the *medialis*, and the *intermedius*—collectively known as the *quadriceps muscle group* of anterior thigh muscles. These chiefly extend the leg. A fifth anterior thigh muscle, the *sartorius*, rotates our entire leg out. This controls the part of the heel bone that will strike the ground when we walk.

The five medial, or inside, muscles of the thigh—*pectineus*, *gracilis*, *adductor longus*, *adductor brevis*, and *adductor magnus*—flex the leg toward the chest and rotate the entire leg inward to control and balance the outward rotation created by the sartorius.

Three muscles at the back of the thigh, the *biceps femoris* or hamstrings, flex the leg (draw the heel toward the buttocks) and extend the thigh (pull the knee away from the chest) to balance the pull of the anterior or front leg muscles.

Again, three groups of muscles control the lower leg. The four anterior muscles lift the foot up away from the ground; they are attached in the foot, mostly by the toes. The two lateral or outside muscles pull the foot toward the ground as well as lifting the outside of the foot away from the ground. The last group of rear leg muscles, in the calf, pull the foot down toward the ground or point the toes.

There are eleven muscles in the foot itself. As with the muscles of the legs, they balance each other on the top, bottom, and sides of the feet, lifting, lowering and twisting the different parts of the feet.

The grand total of muscles in the foot and leg, then, reaches thirty-eight. However, ten muscles in the buttocks and three more in the groin area exert an influence on the movement of the leg. And the muscles of the entire body interact to control the motions of the feet and legs, in an intricate network of checks and balances.

## CIRCULATION

The central organ of the circulatory system is the heart, which pumps blood through the body. Blood is oxygenated by the lungs and then travels to the limbs in arteries. The blood to the feet and legs is carried through the abdominal aorta, which branches out at the groin into two femoral arteries, one for each leg.

The *arteries* are hollow, elastic and muscular tubes. In the foot and leg the major arteries are: the *femoral artery* in the thigh; the *popliteal*, behind the knee; the *anterior tibial*, in the front of the lower leg; the *posterior tibial*, behind the lower leg; the *dorsal pedis*, on top of the foot; and the *medial* and *lateral plantars*, under the foot. The largest arteries have very thick walls and are mostly made up of elastic tissue. The smaller arteries that branch off from these are mostly muscular, helping to keep the blood circulating vigorously. The next smaller branches, the *arterioles*, also contain muscle tissue but have thinner walls.

The *capillaries*, the smallest vessels, actually supply the oxygen and nourishment from the blood to the tissues and absorb waste products to be carried away in the veins. Capillaries have linings which are only one cell thick, so that oxygen and nutrients can easily be exchanged with waste products. All of the nerve endings and hair follicles in the skin are supplied with nutrients by the capillaries. They are extremely sensitive to temperature changes, dilating to allow heat to escape or contracting to conserve it; alcohol and nicotine also affect the capillaries strongly.

The *veins* collect the blood, with its metabolic waste products, from the capillaries and carry it back up toward the heart to be reoxygenated. The veins are elastic tubes, with thinner walls than in the arteries and without muscle tissue. They contain valves which prevent the blood—which is now flowing against gravity—from backing up or flowing back down. Although the veins do not themselves contain muscular tissue, the muscles which they travel through help to push the blood back up toward the heart, since the valves will only allow it to travel upward. The major veins from the foot up to the hip are: the *medial* and *lateral plantar* veins under the feet; the *dorsal venous rete* on top of the foot; the long and short *saphenous* veins near the surface of the lower leg, and their tributaries; the anterior and posterior *tibial* veins in the deep venous system of the lower leg; the *popliteal* vein behind the knee; and, finally, the *femoral* vein in the thigh, extending to the groin. From the lower body the blood travels back to the heart via the *inferior vena cava*.

The *lymphatic system* bathes each of our cells continually. Lymph fluid keeps our tissues hydrated and can help fight local infections. It collects around cells and, in the foot and leg, is supplied and drained by lymph capillaries which lead, by way of superficial (surface) or deep lymph vessels, to or from the *inguinal lymph nodes* of the groin.

## THE NERVES

All the nerves in the feet and legs originate in the lumbar and sacral vertebra at the lower end of the spine. The motor nerves ferry their instructions to the muscles *from* this point; the sensory nerves carry information (heat, pain, texture) back *to* the spine, from where it is relayed up to the brain to be processed and acted on.

We will only mention a few of the most important nerves in the foot and leg here. The *femoral nerve* supplies most of the thigh; the *saphenous, tibial,* and *peroneal* nerves supply the lower leg; the *siatic, sural, medial* and *lateral plantar* nerves supply the bottom of the foot; and the medial and lateral terminal branches of the deep *peroneal* nerve, the top of the foot.

This brief overview is intended to give you a framework by which you can more easily see the interrelationships between the skeletal, muscular, circulatory, and nervous systems of the foot and leg. Keep this interdependency in mind as we discuss the diseases and injuries which can affect the balance between systems in the chapters to come. Pain transferred through the nervous system can cause muscles to tense and shorten, putting strain on ligaments and throwing the skeletal framework out of alignment. Poor circulation can result in muscle cramps or tingling nerves; in the other direction, inactivity and muscle weakness makes it more difficult for the veins to carry blood back up to the heart. The capillaries react to information from the nerve endings, which they feed. These few examples should be enough to demonstrate that in treating problems in the foot and leg it is futile to consider only the muscles, or the bones, or any one system or part. All are interdependent; the goal must be to reestablish their essential balance and harmony.

# Appendix B:
# HERBAL SALVE
# AND SOLUTION

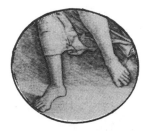

### HERBAL SALVE #1

1 qt. cold-pressed safflower, sunflower,
  or canola oil.
½ oz. comfrey leaves
½ oz. goldenseal root
½ oz. peppermint leaves
Vitamin E (d-alpha tocopherol) capsules
Vitamin A (B-carotene) capsules
Vitamin D capsules from a vegetable-
  derived source
Mason jar, of the type used to put up
  preserves
Cheesecloth

Mix the oil, comfrey leaves, goldenseal root, and peppermint
leaves in a large pot—an electric pot is excellent. Heat the
mixture at a *very* low temperature. You must be able to test
the oil by placing your finger in it without burning yourself.
The oil should only be warm, never hot (approximately 150°
Fahrenheit). Start this process early in the morning as you
must allow the mixture to "cook" for at least twelve to
twenty-four hours. The purpose of this procedure is to leach
out the natural herbal healing agents without destroying
them with excessive heat. Cold-pressed oil is best because it
contains vitamins, such as vitamin E, and minerals which help

in healing and can be destroyed in extraction processes that use high heat. After the oil has been "cooked," strain it through clean, fresh cheesecloth (you can boil it first to kill bacteria) twice to remove impurities that could become abrasive to inflamed or damaged skin. Add to this the contents of the vitamin capsules.

It is wise to add at least 25,000 to 50,000 IU of each vitamin. You can pop open the capsules using a round toothpick. Mix the vitamins in well with the oil. Note that the oil will probably have taken on a green color from the herbs during the cooking process.

If the salve is kept refrigerated in the mason jar it will last for up to 6 months. The vitamin E in the oil and from the capsules will help act as a natural preservative. It is a good idea to buy a small ointment jar from the pharmacy or health-food store which can hold half an ounce or one ounce of salve. Thus a small amount of salve can be kept at room temperature for daily use and the rest refrigerated to maintain its potency.

The salve must be used three times a day. Gently rub in a small amount. Wipe away any excess salve that doesn't absorb into the skin. Discontinue use if skin irritation develops. This antifungal, antibacterial salve is ideal for fungus infections, cuts, scratches, bee stings, and so on; but never use it on deep wounds or cuts, nor around the eyes. Yes, it is safe to eat a little by mistake! You may reduce the ingredients proportionately to reduce costs.

## HERBAL SOLUTION #1

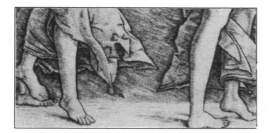

1 qt. boiled water
¼ oz. comfrey leaves
¼ oz. goldenseal root
¼ oz. peppermint leaves
1-quart mason jar
Cheesecloth

Make a tea by adding the ingredients to the boiling water. Allow the mixture to stand, covered, for thirty minutes. Carefully strain the solution with the cheesecloth twice, to remove all the leaves. Allow the solution to cool at room temperature; never use it boiling hot. The solution may be kept in a closed jar for forty-eight hours before being discarded. The amount of ingredients may be reduced proportionately to lower cost.

Wrap the area to be treated with sterile gauze or bandage. Pour just enough of the solution onto the gauze to thoroughly saturate it. Allow the gauze to completely air-dry. Repeat the process as often as necessary.

This solution is antifungal, antibacterial, and mildly astringent. Used as described above, it acts like a poultice. It will help bring infections in the skin to a head, reduce itching and inflammation in the skin, and dry up oozing skin problems caused by abrasions of the skin, fungus infections, and so on. Never soak your feet in a basin of the solution, and discontinue use of the solution if skin irritation occurs.

# Appendix C:
# SUPPLIERS

Most foot specialists have a relationship with one manufacturer of orthotics, and will recommend that company's wares to their patients. These companies are all reputable and their products comparable.

The shoe that best fits your foot and needs should ideally be found in a well-stocked sports shoe store, where you can compare many brands and styles. The sales people in these stores are usually trustworthy and know their merchandise well. Their advice coupled with the recommendations given in Chapter 7 should ensure that you end up with the right shoe. Your needs will be very individual, and it is pointless here to endorse one particular brand of shoe as best for everyone. However, the names and addresses of those companies that make shoes in unusual widths may be useful to those who live in small communities where the range in their local stores may be limited, especially in wide or narrow sizes. These companies are:

**FOR NARROW FEET:**

Brooks Shoe Inc.
131 Factory Street
Hanover, Penn. 17331
(717) 632-1755

## FOR WIDE AND NARROW FEET:

New Balance Athletic Shoes
38 Everett Street
Boston, Mass. 02134
(617) 783-4000

Van Doren Rubber Company (makers of Vans shoes)
2095 Batavia Street
Orange, Calif. 92665
(714) 974-7414

## AND FOR WIDE FEET:

Hyde Athletic Industries (makers of Saucony shoes)
Box 6046
Peabody, Mass. 01961
(617) 532-9000

## THE MANUFACTURERS OF SUPPORT STOCKINGS
## FOR VARICOSE VEINS MENTIONED IN CHAPTER 3 ARE:

Becton, Dickinson and Co. (Bauer & Black stockings)
1 Becton Drive
Franklin Lakes, N.J. 07417

The Kendall Co.
1 Federal Street
Boston, Mass. 02101
(617) 423-2000

Parke, Davis and Co.
Box 1510
Rochester, Mich. 48063
(313) 651-9081

## FOR CUSTOM-MADE SUPPORT STOCKINGS:

Jobst Institute Inc.
653 Miami Street
Toledo, Ohio 43605
(419) 698-1611

Sigvaris, Inc.
32 Park Drive East
Branford, CT 06405-6545
(203) 481-5588

**COMPANIES MENTIONED IN CHAPTER 7
THAT MAKE ORTHOTICS:**

Langer Biomechanics Group Inc.
21 East Industry Court
Deer Park, N.Y. 11729
(516) 667-3042

Spenco Medical Corp.
Box 2501
Waco, Tex. 76702
(817) 772-6000

# GLOSSARY

**accessory bones**  Two small, round bones found under the ball of the foot (the end of the first metatarsal bone) in everyone.

**achilles tendon**  The tendon formed from the calf muscles (soleus, gastrocnemius) attached to the heel bone (calcaneus) behind the ankle.

**acupressure**  Deep, forceful pressure applied to areas on the body (usually related to acupuncture meridian points, or trigger points) for healing purposes.

**acute**  Severe and characterized by swift onset. Used in the description of injury symptoms such as pain, or the course of disease.

**adhesions**  Fibrous strands of tissue that form internally in a specific anatomical region following injury or surgery.

**aerobic exercise**  Any exercise that uses major muscle groups in a rhythmic and continuous way.

**antihistamines**  A group of naturally occurring chemicals in the body that stop the symptoms produced by the action of histamine (allergy symptoms).

**arch**  in the feet, the curved appearance of the bone structure in normal feet.

**artery**  A hollow tube carrying blood away from the heart to every cell in the body.

159

**athlete's foot**   A common layperson's term to describe any fungus infection in the skin of the feet.

**belladonna foods**   Foods that contain the naturally occurring substance atropine alkaloid, such as tomatoes, yellow onions, white potatoes, peppers, and eggplant.

**bone spur**   A sharp projection of bone formed by additional layers of calcium over a site fracture, stress fracture, or because of repeated, excessive pressure.

**bowlegs**   The common name for *Genu varum,* which is an outward bowing of the legs.

**bunion**   The bump or enlargement of the head of the first metatarsal bone of the side of the foot.

**calcaneus**   The heel bone.

**callus**   Thickened, hard, dry skin over a diffuse area under the foot caused by excessive friction or intermittent pressure from exercise, ill-fitting shoes, abnormal bones or ground pressure.

**capillary**   The smallest blood vessel uniting the arterial and venous blood circulation.

**chronic**   Said of an injury or disease of long duration, slow development or recurring, often mild, symptoms.

**claudication pains**   Cramping pains in legs caused by a lack of arterial blood flowing into muscles and build-up of muscle cell waste products.

**clubfoot**   Any deformity involving the talus bone in the foot, causing abnormal twisted positions of the foot.

**cold-pressed**   Said of an oil derived by squeezing the fruit, nut or seed, without the use of heat which destroys natural vitamins found in the oil.

**combination lasts**   The mold on which various kinds of shoes can be constructed, using a wider front area and a narrower heel area.

**counter**   A support, usually made of leather or plastic, which is built into the rear portion of a shoe.

**cuboid**   A bone found in the middle of the foot, cube-like in shape.

**cuneiform**   Three small, wedge-shaped bones found in the middle of the foot.

**dermatitis**   An inflammation of any kind in the skin, characterized by itching, scaling, oozing or eruptions.

**drop foot**   Usually a symptom of neurological damage from stroke, accident or disease. Drop foot renders dorsiflexion, the raising the foot upwards towards the shin when walking, impossible.

**earth shoe**   A type of shoe made in the 1970s, that positions the heel lower than the sole. It can produce strain on the calf muscle during walking.

**edema**   Swelling of the feet and legs with water.

**electrodessication**   The use of electric current to destroy abnormal tissue, such as warts.

**endorphin**   Naturally occurring chemicals in the brain which control pain and which have been linked to the "runner's high" felt after any aerobic exercising.

**femoral nerve**   A nerve which originates in the second, third and fourth lumbar nerves to supply the skin and muscles of the front of the thigh.

**femur**   The thigh bone.

**fibula**   The long bone on the outer side of the lower leg.

**fissures**   Deep cracks in the skin, often caused by fungus infections.

**flared heel**   A heel on a shoe that is wider than the upper part of the shoe, giving additional medial and lateral stability to the ankle and the foot.

**flat-footed**   A condition wherein the arch of the foot collapses with each step (see *pes planus*).

**ganglionic cyst**   An abnormal sac attached to the lining of a tendon, containing a thick, extremely viscous (jelly-like) fluid comprised of mucopolysaccharides and fibrous tissue. Ganglionic cysts usually occur on the feet or hands.

**gastrocnemius**   A muscle of the rear lower leg. The gastrocnemius arises from the lower back portion of the femur, extends down the center of the calf to the center portion of the achilles tendon, and finally attaches to the rear of the heel bone. Its main purpose is to lift the heel and propel it forward during ambulation (walking).

**gout**   An inherited condition in which the body is unable to eliminate purines (protein metabolism waste products such as uric acid), causing acute joint pain as well as other longer lasting symptoms.

**hammer toes**   A congenital abnormality in which toes are flexed at the first toe joint. The condition may or may not involve pain; the toes may or may not be rigid.

**hamstring**   Either of two groups of tendons bounding the upper part of the popliteal space at the back of the knee and forming the tendons of insertion of certain muscles of the back of the thigh.

**hemosiderin**   A golden yellow or yellow-brown product of digestion of iron which turns red brown when oxidized.

**hemosiderin deposits**   Redish-brown color change in the lower leg caused by passage of hemosiderin through the blood vessel walls into the fat and subcutaneous tissues of the legs and feet.

**homans' sign**   Pain in the calf in response to gentle squeezing or upward flexion (dorsiflexion). It is indicative of incipient or established thrombosis (clotting) in the veins of the leg.

**ileotibial band syndrome**   Inflammation of a fibrous tissue which extends from the crest of the ilium (the broad, flaring portion of the hip bone) to the tibia's lateral condyle (the outside portion of the thigh bone), due to upper and lower body imbalances.

**impetigo**   A bacterial infection of the skin that is very contagious.

**in-toeing**   An abnormal turning inward of the foot and leg while walking, commonly called 'pigeon-toed' walking.

**incompetent valves**   These are abnormal, tissue-like 'gates' in veins which allow blood backflow, causing blood clots, phlebitis, varicose skin, ulcers and infections.

**inguinal lymph nodes**  Numerous large, circular masses found in the upper inner thigh region of the groin. They collect the lymph from the leg.

**knock-kneed**  When the thigh bone in-curves excessively, such that the knees touch or almost touch. The opposite of bowlegged.

**ligament**  A fibrous band of tissue attached to two or more bones inside and/or outside a joint, stablizing it and permitting controlled movement.

**lumbar vertebrae**  The five vertebrae, or backbones, found in the lower back above the sacral backbones and beneath the thoracic backbones. Most of the nerves to the feet and legs arise from the lumbar vertebrae.

**lymph**  A clear, transparent, sometimes faintly yellow fluid that is collected from the cells of the body, transported through the lymphatic system, and eventually added to the venous blood circulation. Lymph consists of a clear fluid in which can be found varying numbers of white blood cells and a few red blood cells.

**lymphatic systems**  The network of lymph vessels, nodes, etc., which carry the lymph fluid to and from the cells.

**march fracture**  The common name given to stress fractures of the metatarsal bones in the feet.

**metabolic wastes**  The end product of all forms of metabolism in the body.

**metatarsal joints**  The joints found at the distal (towards the toes) end of the metatarsal bones of the foot.

**metatarsus adductus**  An abnormal, inward (towards the center of the body) deviation of the metatarsal bones of the foot.

**midsole**  The portion of a shoe between the upper portion and the outersole which touches the ground.

**multidirectional**  Able to move in many or all directions.

**navicular**  A major bone of the rear foot, found next to the cuboid bone in front of the talus bone and behind the first and second cuneiform bones.

**nevus** A birthmark, usually circular, commonly called a 'beauty mark.' Nevi may be brown, black or red.

**nicotine** A chemical found naturally in tobacco of all kinds. Among its properties is that it causes blood vessels in the hands, feet and skin to close temporarily.

**nightbar** Also called 'nightsplint.' Layperson's term for a Dennis-Browne bar which is attached to the sole of baby shoes to correct abnormal positions of the thigh bones (e.g., intoeing or out-toeing). It consists of a rigid strip of aluminum or steel alloy.

**noninvasive** Any therapy, treatment or test which does not involve penetration of the body.


**optimum heart rate** The ideal heart rate at rest or during exercise. Ideal heart rates will vary from person to person.

**Orlon** A man-made material used in socks and various clothes items. It is a lightweight material, but doesn't 'breathe' to allow perspiration to be released.

**orthopedic** Having to do with the development and treatment of bones.

**orthotic** Referring to a biomechanical device which is worn inside shoes to maintain the integrity of the bones of the foot during ambulation (walking) by allowing only normal ranges of motion of joints and bones. A variety of materials may be used in the manufacture of orthotic devices.

**osteoarthritis** A condition or disease affecting the joints. Recent studies point to the presence of an 'overactive' immune system as being a prominent causal factor.

**osteoporosis** A condition wherein calcium is leached from bones into the blood stream, reducing the overall quantity of bone mass and causing many symptoms including but not limited to pain and spontaneous bone fractures. Typically, osteoporosis occurs in postmenopausal women and elderly men.

**out-toeing** An abnormal twisting outward of the feet and legs when walking.


**patella** The bone of the knee cap.

**periostitis** An inflammation, often very painful, of the

micro-thin lining of the outside of any bone (the periosteum).

**pes planus**   Permanent collapse of the arch of the foot.

**phlebitis**   An inflammation of a vein caused by a blood clot
(thrombus) or a marked slowing of the venous blood flow.

**plantar wart**   A virus-induced, often painful tumor found on
the sole of the foot.

**plantar fascia**   A band of muscle found under the foot in the
arch area. It extends from the front of the heel to the
metatarsal bones.

**plantar fascitis**   An inflammation of the plantar fascia musculature causing pain and muscle spasm, often mistaken for
stress fracture of the heel bone.

**podiatrist**   A doctor who has specialized in the study and
treatment of foot and leg problems.

**polypropylene**   A synthetic fiber used in various clothing to
help draw perspiration away from the skin.

**popliteal artery**   The main artery found directly behind the
knee, beginning at the end of the femoral artery of the
thigh and ending shortly in the common peroneal artery of
the lower leg. This artery feeds all the structures in and
around the knee.

**poultice**   Any material applied to the body that effects a
healing action through evaporation and/or a transfer of
medicinal agents into the skin (e.g., a poultice containing
wet moss or mud for a bee sting). Poultices are often applied hot.

**pronation**   A turning inward and downward of some of the
bones in and around the ankle joints. Normal pronation is a
natural movement of the foot during the first fifteen percent of each step when walking and may be considered an
adaptive motion of the foot to the ground. Excessive pronation is the number one cause of a majority of mechanical
foot complaints and injuries.

**psoriasis**   A skin condition caused by emotional or nutritional stress. Psoriasis appears as dry, peely, itchy, inflamed, silvery-scaled skin.

**purines**   Naturally occurring component substances which
may lead to gout in some people who don't eliminate them

properly from the blood. Purines are found in high levels in the following foods: meat and organ foods, whole grains, spinach, watercress, mushrooms, peas, lima beans, lentils, onions, alcohol, tea and coffee.

**rheumatoid arthritis**   An often severe form of arthritis, seen in women more than men. Typically, the onset of rheumatoid arthritis occurs during the person's mid-thirties. It is characterized by severe pain, stiffness and deformity of joints, worsening over time.

**sacral vertebrae**   The five sacral vertebrae contain nerves that effect the legs and buttock area. Found just below the five lumbar vertebrae and just above the tail bone, the sacral vertebrae appear to be fused together.

**saphenous nerve**   Extending from the femoral nerve near the groin to the feet, the saphenous nerve supplies the nerves to the skin of the feet and legs.

**serotonin**   A vasoconstrictor (causing constriction of our blood vessels) which is present in relatively high concentrations in some areas of the central nervous system and in many peripheral tissues.

**shiatsu**   A deep body massage technique that is actually a variation of acupuncture developed by the Japanese. In shiatsu, deep pressure is applied to specific points on our body by the fingers, knuckles, elbows and knees.

**shin splints**   Injury to and inflammation of the muscles in the front of the leg. Shin splints cause the muscles to pull away from the bone, causing inflammation and leading to pain and tenderness of the affected area.

**soleus**   A broad flat muscle of the calf which lifts the heel up off of the ground. The soleus is on the inner and outer side of the rear lower leg starting at the upper portions of the tibia and fibula bones near the knee and extending down to the rear of the heel bone, where it becomes part of the achilles tendon.

**sprain**   An injury to a ligament when the joint is carried through a range of motion greater than normal, but without dislocation or fracture.

**stress fracture**   A fracture of bone caused by sudden force, or repeated force beyond the bone's tolerance. Often, stress fractures involve imbalances of foot structure and/or upper body structure.

**subacute**   Between acute and chronic, denoting the course of a disease or injury.

**synovial fluid**   A liquid substance manufactured by synovial membrane and found in joints. Synovial fluid, also called synovia, serves as a lubricant to reduce friction and wear on the joints.

**synovial membrane**   A tissue that lines the synovial joints, but does not cover cartilage, and which produces synovial fluid.

**talus**   One of the ankle bones. The talus sits over the heel bone and between the malleoli (the bones on either side of the ankle joint at the end portion of the fibula and tibia bones).

**tendon**   A fibrous part of a muscle which attaches to a bone to produce movement when the muscle contracts.

**tendonitis**   An inflammation of part or all of the tendonous portion of a muscle due to injury or disease, causing pain, swelling and muscle spasm.

**thermoplastic**   A heat-moldable plastic used in orthotic manufacturing.

**thrombophlebitis**   An inflammation in a vein caused by a blood cot.

**tibia**   The larger, thicker, wider lower leg bone.

**toe clips**   Can be used on bicycle pedals to clamp shoes to pedals during biking.

**triathlete**   A person who trains and participates in three events or races in one competition.

**ulcer**   A sore or wound of the skin with loss of tissue with or without infection.

**unidirectional**   Movement in one direction only.

**uric acid**   The dissolved crystals found in blood and urine which can cause pain in joints in gout. Uric acid may also form stones in the bladder or kidneys, producing a variety of health complaints.

**varicose veins**   Veins that have dilated (enlarged) due to improper closure of the valves inside them.

**vasoconstrictor**   Any drug or other agent that causes arteries to close.

**vasodilator**   Any drug or other agent that causes arteries to open.

**vasospasm**   A constriction of the muscular portions of an artery causing partial or complete closure.

**vein**   A blood vessel that brings blood back to the heart.

Nonfiction from **Four Walls Eight Windows**

Bachmann, Steve.
**Preach Liberty: Selections from the Bible for Progressives.** pb: $10.95.

David, Kati.
**A Child's War: World War II Through the Eyes of Children.** cl: $17.95.

Dubuffet, Jean.
**Asphyxiating Culture and Other Writings.** cl: $17.95.

Gould, Jay, and Goldman, Benjamin.
**Deadly Deceit: Low-Level Radiation, High-Level Cover-Up.** cl: $19.95.

Hoffman, Abbie.
**The Best of Abbie Hoffman: Selections from
"Revolution for the Hell of It," "Woodstock Nation,"
"Steal this Book," and New Writings.** cl: $21.95.

Johnson, Phyllis, and Martin, David, eds.
**Frontline Southern Africa: Destructive Engagement.** cl: $23.95, pb: $14.95.

Jones, E.P.
**Where Is Home? Living Through Foster Care.** cl: $17.95.

Wasserman, Harvey.
**Harvey Wasserman's History of the United States.** pb: $8.95.

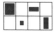

Fiction from **Four Walls Eight Windows**

Algren, Nelson.
**The Man with the Golden Arm.** pb: $9.95.

Algren, Nelson.
**Never Come Morning.** pb: $8.95.

Algren, Nelson.
**The Neon Wilderness.** pb: $7.95.

Anderson, Sherwood.
**The Triumph of the Egg.** pb: $8.95.

Boetie, Dugmore.
**Familiarity Is the Kingdom of the Lost.** pb: $6.95.

Brodsky, Michael.
**Dyad.** cl: $23.95, pb: $11.95.

Brodsky, Michael.
**Xman.** cl: $21.95, pb.$11.95.

Brodsky, Michael.
**X in Paris.** pb: $9.95.

Codrescu, Andrei, ed.
**American Poetry Since 1970: Up Late,** 2nd ed. pb: $14.95.

Grimes, Tom.
**A Stone of the Heart.** cl: $15.95.

Howard-Howard, Margo (with Abbe Michaels).
**I Was a White Slave in Harlem.** pb: $10.95.

Martin, Augustine, ed.
**Forgiveness: Ireland's Best Contemporary
Short Stories.** cl: $25.95, pb: $12.95.

Santos, Rosario, ed.
**And We Sold the Rain: Contemporary Fiction
from Central America.** cl: $18.95, pb: $9.95.

Sokolov, Sasha. **A School for Fools.** pb: $9.95.

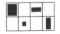

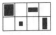

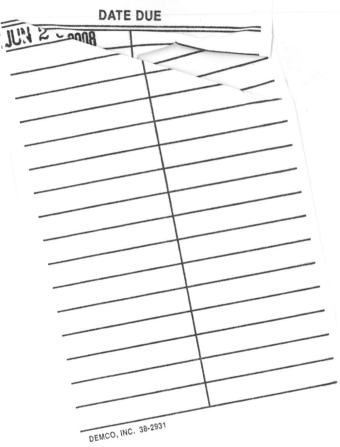

DATE DUE

JUN 2 2008

DEMCO, INC. 38-2931